Diet and Cancer:

Is There a Connection?

Health Secrets to Slowing Cancer If You Have It & Preventing Cancer If You Don't

with Splash!

WHAT EVERY WOMAN SHOULD KNOW!

Diet and Cancer:

Is There a Connection?

Health Secrets to Slowing Cancer If You Have It & Preventing Cancer If You Don't

©2010, Melinda Coker
with Splash! LLC
http://www.DietCancerConnection.com

with Splash!

In Loving Memory

Sara Nan Chamberlain Quiroz
February 25, 1950 – April 17, 2007

Betty Marie Earnest Danielson
November 14, 1943 – October 25, 2009

Bunker's "Pogo" Coker
February 17, 2000 – September 14, 2009

Acknowledgments

With all my love to my sweet, kind, and enduringly patient husband, who has supported me wholeheartedly in my research and writing of this book.

Contents

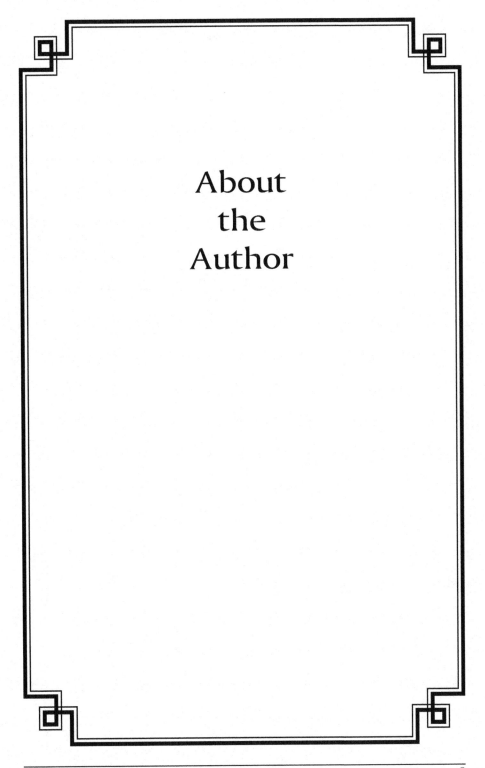

About
the
Author

Melinda Coker is a health coach and consultant who has studied and researched health and wellness issues for over 30 years. She helps clients develop healthy habits to repair their bodies and achieve a renewed feeling of well-being.

As a licensed counselor, Melinda has worked with hundreds of clients, helping them gain the skills needed to improve their lives. She is a passionate researcher of health information and truly believes that we can prevent many of the major diseases that affect our lives and the lives of our families. She has practiced healthy living for years, and has affectionately been called a "health nut" by her many friends.

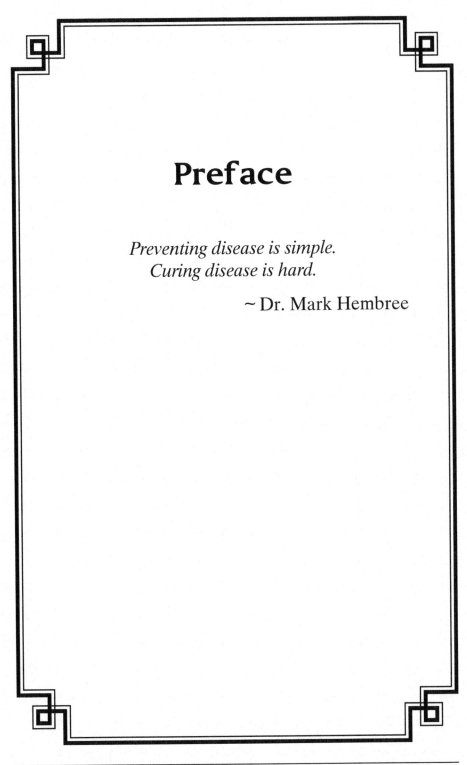

Preface

Preventing disease is simple.
Curing disease is hard.

~ Dr. Mark Hembree

I have recently lost two good friends to cancer. They were beautiful women in the prime of life who made the world a better place for their families and friends. Then they were gone.

My world changed that summer day in 2004 when I learned of my friend Nan's cancer diagnosis. I couldn't believe it. Cancer was supposed to happen to "old" people or people you didn't really know, but it certainly wasn't supposed to happen to a good friend who seemed perfectly healthy.

Since that summer, many other friends have been diagnosed with cancer and have suffered through treatments. Too many people are affected, and I want to help in some way.

I'm not good at holding hands while someone vomits, but I can research ways to help people prevent cancer and give those already diagnosed a way to improve their odds, thus giving them more time to live and to spend with their families and their precious children and grandchildren.

I've been interested in living a healthy lifestyle for nearly 40 years. A major turning point occurred during my husband's years in dental school, when I learned that tooth decay was truly preventable.

After suffering at the hands of a dentist who filled my cavities without deadening shots or nitrous oxide, this was truly an amazing concept. Decay was caused by sugar and bacteria, and not just because you had "soft" teeth. You mean you could eliminate candies and sodas and brush your teeth after meals and before bed and you could actually grow up without fillings? Why hadn't I known that?

I am a rabid reader and have always had my nose stuck in a book. Most of my reading is nonfiction on how to "better" my life; whether through exercise, cooking, being a mother, or studying any health-related topic. After all, if there was a way we could eliminate tooth decay on our own, there was probably a way to eliminate many other ailments and diseases.

I have listened to lectures, and read hundreds of books and articles. It seems that the more I read, the more confused I got. I tried to follow the rules, but there were new and sometimes contradictory rules coming out every day. In fact, over the years my family has endured more "diets" than most people have socks!

Concentrating and learning about cancer has developed my focus and made me more determined to follow my plan without getting bounced all over the place from conflicting views and opinions. Through this book, I want to help you "cut out the clutter" so you too can focus on what's important.

Some of you may ask, "How will the advice in this book differ from that offered in other health books—those written by doctors and nutritionists and cancer patients and survivors?"

This book is primarily for those women looking to protect themselves and their families from cancer and other major health problems through lifestyle choices. You will learn what I learned from over 30 years of asking questions and searching for answers.

As we age, our chance of getting cancer increases. There may not be a way to totally stop us from getting it, but if I can have a 50% chance of avoiding it, you'd better know that I'll take it.

I am not a doctor. I am not a scientist. But I am an advocate of learning all I can about health and the prevention of disease, and then putting those practices into effect in my own life. As my relatives and friends know, I often try to get others to put those same practices into their lives as well.

If you want to protect your family from the horrors of cancer, this book is for you. It might even save your life.

Introduction

*Just about everything worth doing is
worth doing because it's important
and because the odds are against you.
If they weren't,
then anyone could do it,
so don't bother.*

~Seth Godin

Cancer sucks.

It turns lives upside down. It turns people into patients. It causes doctors to hurriedly recommend terrible treatments for their new patients to endure. Families become traumatized, schedules become upended, and the costs can become exorbitant even with insurance.

Before beginning my research into cancer, I thought it was just a big, scary, random disease that we got through "the luck of the draw." As I have learned more and more about the causes and the growth of the disease, it has become less frightening because I have read statistics that say from 40%–70% of cancers are actually preventable. The odds of keeping cancer at bay have gotten a whole lot better.

One of the most important books I have read was *The China Study*.[1] Soon after reading that, I recommended it to numerous friends and acquaintances—but they didn't read it. I was disappointed and tried to think of other ways to get this important information into the hands of my friends.

That's when I decided to write my own book. Maybe if I were the author, I would have more impact in getting them to read it. If I can have an impact and save even one person's life with the information in this book, it will have been worth the exorbitant amount of energy and hard work it has taken to put it together. Here's a brief overview of what you will learn as you read the book.

Your Odds of Getting a Cancer Diagnosis

Over 1,500 Americans die of cancer every day. One in two of us will be diagnosed with cancer in our lifetime. We have spent billions of dollars on cancer research, yet the numbers keep going up. In Chapter 1, you will learn that we need to intervene earlier or learn to prevent cancer in the first place.

What Exactly Is Cancer?

Cancer is considered a progressive disease and can grow inside our bodies for years or even decades. We get abnormal changes in the DNA of our genes on a regular basis, but many times the genes can be repaired. However, if not repaired, the damaged genes can go on to eventually become cancer.

In Chapter 2, you will learn about the three stages of cancer. Mammograms usually don't pick up breast cancer until the cancer cells have been growing for 14 years, so during all the years of the second stage, you can do things to slow down the growth, speed it up, or possibly even stop it.

What Are Some Risk Factors for the Different Types of Cancer?

Chapter 3 is organized into a list of the 21 most common cancers, and describes the currently known risk factors for each type. Many of the risk factors on the list seem to cause specific tumor cells to grow. For example, if you are a smoker, you will most likely get damaged cells in your lungs or your esophagus.

What Are Some General Risk Factors for Cancer?

If we are continually being bombarded with risks, why don't we individually have multiple cancers being diagnosed at any one time in our lives? I don't think we truly know the answer to that question yet, but we do know that our bodies can repair many of those genes which have mutated.

It could depend on the health of our immune system at the time of exposure. It could depend on our genetics. If we have certain genes and we are then exposed to a certain risk, that could cause the mutation to continue to grow. Chapter 4 lists 33 of the most common cancer risk factors by type of hazard.

Early Detection or Prevention?

Because cancers take so long to grow before we can detect them, counting on "early detection" can kill us. We need to think about prevention. In Chapter 5, you will learn that there are numerous research studies which show that, if all of us choose our diet carefully, we can make a huge difference in the number of cancers diagnosed and the number of people dying from cancer.

How Can You Prevent Cancer?

The first step would obviously be to make sure you are not exposed to any risks, and that your body and your immune system are in top-notch condition so you can fight off any of the demons that try to catch you.

Are there other steps you can take? Many dermatologists think that if you apply enough sunscreen or stay out of the sun entirely, you can avoid melanomas and other skin cancers. If you avoid smoking and all tobacco products and all second-hand smoke, you may be able to avoid lung cancer.

If our chemotherapy and radiation treatments aren't working to keep our cancer patients alive, why not try something else? Chapter 6 gives a list of lifestyle changes that could make a difference.

Should I Change the Way I Live?

Changing your lifestyle is never easy, but it can be done just like bad habits can be replaced with good ones. We have all done it. Chapter 7 will explain how to make it work.

Lifestyle Myths

Chapter 8 will give you the answers to the numerous questions you will be asked once you announce that you are changing your lifestyle.

A Road Map for Change

Once you decide to change, you may want a plan to get you started. In Chapter 9, I give you a 10-day plan for beginning healthy eating habits.

By the time you finish this book, I hope you will have a clearer view of the research and scientific writings about the connection that your diet has with cancer, and I hope you will have learned that you can increase your chances of living a long, full, healthy, and cancer-free life.

This book is intended for informational purposes only, and should not be interpreted as specific medical advice. You should consult with a qualified health care provider for medical advice and diagnosis, or if you are experiencing any acute or specific health concerns.

Chapter 1:
A Cancer Diagnosis

*But when I first got cancer, after the
initial shock and the fear
and paranoia and crying
and all that goes with cancer - that word
means to most people ultimate death -
I decided to see what I could do
to take that negative
and use it in a positive way.*

~ Herbie Mann

Cancer seems so random to us. People with no apparent genetic link are suddenly diagnosed. People who seem to be in excellent health are suddenly diagnosed. We hear, "Well, he ate a really good diet and he exercised, and he died of cancer."

"When the doctor told me I had cancer, my life as I knew it came to a screeching halt," recalls my friend Paula, a 56-year-old investment banker. "It took nearly four months just to get a diagnosis because everyone kept assuring me that my symptoms were nothing serious.

"When the doctor finally called me back to his office after undergoing another series of tests, I knew it was going to be bad news. When he blurted out that it was cancer, I burst into tears. I couldn't believe it! I do all the right things. I've never smoked, I run four times a week, and I have no family history of cancer. I've basically been in a mental free fall since then.

"The following week was a blur of medical appointments and it was decided that I would have surgery right away.

"The surgery went well, but at my first post-op appointment I learned that there were signs the cancer had spread. Once again, I was plunged into despair. I then consulted three oncologists and opted for radiation therapy. I had to go to the hospital for a 15-minute treatment every day for weeks.

"I work long hours because work is the only thing that keeps me sane. It's when I'm away from work that the problems start to overwhelm me. Sometimes I feel like I'm drowning and it's hard to stay hopeful. I've become irritable and argumentative, but I'm angry. Why me? Why now? Why didn't I find another doctor?

"On my good days, I am determined to survive this disease. Unfortunately, I have a lot of bad days, too. There are some nights when I lie awake, terrified that I'll die or become so sick that I'll be a burden to my family.

"In our society, sick people are constantly urged to 'be positive' and those of us who are unable to see the silver lining feel like failures. I want to be strong, but I'm overwhelmed with fear. I can't help thinking, *'What if I die?'*"

Paula's concerns are certainly real. Approximately 562,340 Americans are expected to die of cancer this year.[1] That is over 1,500 a day, equivalent to *three* jumbo jets (which hold 400–500 people) crashing and killing everyone on board every day of the year.[2]

Cancer is the second most common cause of death in the U.S., exceeded only by heart disease.[3]

During the four to six years of World War II, nearly 500,000 Americans died in what is considered the deadliest military conflict in history; yet cancer can kill even more Americans in only one year.

Another 1.47 million[4] will learn of their cancer diagnosis this year when they have that "most frightening of conversations" with their doctor.[5] One veteran cancer researcher sums it up by declaring, "It is as if one World Trade Center tower were collapsing on our society every single day."[6]

One in two men and women will be diagnosed with cancer during their lifetime.[7]

These stark numbers remind us that we are definitely losing "The War on Cancer" launched by President Nixon in 1971, and that the conventional approaches to treating most cancers have proved to be a stunning failure.

What has happened? We have spent close to $200 billion through taxes, donations, and private funding since 1971 on this "War."[8] According to the National Cancer Institute's online database, there have been 1.56 million papers published about cancer research.[9] With that huge number of scientific experiments reported on, you would think we would be close to a "cure."

Looking at the numbers—of cancer deaths, of cancer diagnoses, and the amount of money we've spent looking for a cure—I think you could say that the United States has a cancer epidemic.

Michael Sporn, a professor of pharmacology and medicine at Dartmouth Medical School, believes that we need to intervene earlier in the process—especially at key points when precancerous lesions occur.[10]

We have been able to prevent millions of heart attacks and strokes by using an early intervention strategy. Heart disease doesn't start with the heart attack; it starts with elevated blood cholesterol and lipids that cause arterial plaque. So we treat those. Stroke doesn't start with the blood clot in the brain. It starts with hypertension. So we treat it with both lifestyle changes and drugs.

A good example of early detection that works is the Pap smear, which detects premalignant changes in the cells of the cervix. That simple procedure, followed by the surgical removal of any lesions, has dropped the incidence and death rates from cervical cancer by 78% since it was developed in the 1950s.[11]

The same goes for colon cancer. Colon cancers have to go through an abnormal step called an adenomatous polyp before becoming deadly. Other precursors to cancer include Barrett's esophagus and hyperkeratosis (head and neck cancers).

A few cancer researchers have made great strides in finding more early warning signs and precancerous conditions. Lance Liotta, chief of pathology at the NCI, has demonstrated that ovarian cancer can be detected by a high-tech blood test, and early results on a protein test for pancreatic cancer are promising as well.[12]

So many people seem to be obsessed with miraculous cures in our "war on cancer" rather than the simple things we can do now such as prevention and early precursors. We used to try to prevent lung cancer with chest x-rays, which was a complete failure. Now we teach people not to smoke.[13]

You may have gone to the doctor because of a vague, minor symptom but, after taking a multitude of tests, you are told you have cancer. That moment in time when you go from being a healthy person with a busy, fulfilling life to a person with cancer is truly dreadful.

Immediately your physicians will want you to begin some form of conventional treatment; surgery, chemotherapy, or radiation. And each decision has to be made in haste, "because we caught it so early," or "we caught it so late," or "it's a very aggressive form of tumor."

Every person you know and love will be affected by cancer, either their own or that of a close friend or family member, so I hope you are ready to learn about it.

Chapter 2:
What Is Cancer and How Does It Start?

Growth for the sake of growth
is the ideology
of the cancer cell.

~ Edward Abbey,
American Author

Cancer is not a disease that you catch like a common cold. You do not get infected and then diagnosed three weeks later. Cancer is a progressive disease with many possible causes.

If we go through a little biology, it may help you visualize the process. Our bodies are made up of cells. Of course we can't count the cells, but there are estimates that we are composed of a hundred trillion cells.[1] Those hundred trillion cells are divided into roughly 320 different types, which include muscle cells, skin cells, and brain cells, among others.[2]

Inside each cell is a nucleus, or a control center. Within that nucleus are 23 pairs of chromosomes; one of each of those pairs comes from your mother and the other from your father. Within each chromosome are hundreds to thousands of genes, and each gene has a DNA sequence made up of molecules.[3]

Abnormal changes in our DNA are called mutations. These mutations in our cells happen all the time, but the cell usually detects the change and repairs it or tells it to die (apoptosis). If the mutation is not repaired, it may lead to the development of cancer.[4]

There are two types of mutations: hereditary and acquired. Hereditary mutations are those passed from parent to child at birth. These mutations are then present in all cells of the child, and can be a factor in 5–10% of all cancers.

Acquired mutations are those DNA changes caused by things in the environment which make a specified cause of the disease hard to determine.[5] Some environmental causes of cancer can include tobacco, chemicals, viruses, radiation, hormones, chronic inflammation, faulty genes, and even the toxins from nuts and seeds. These various carcinogens can genetically transform normal cells into cancer-prone cells by causing damage to the cell's DNA.[6]

Most scientists believe that cancer develops through a process that has more than one mutation, and likely several of them. So if a person inherits a mutation, at least one more mutation is needed to damage the gene enough that it does not function.[7]

The two main types of genes that play a role in cancer are the oncogenes and the tumor suppressor genes. When a proto-oncogene (a good gene) changes into an oncogene, it becomes a bad gene and begins to grow out of control. Think of the proto-oncogene as the gas pedal in your car which regulates how fast the cell grows and divides. In the oncogene, the gas pedal sticks and causes the cell to divide out of control.[8]

The tumor suppressor genes are normal genes that can slow down cell division, repair DNA mistakes, or tell cells when to die (apoptosis). We can think of tumor suppressor genes as the brake pedal in a car, slowing down the process and keeping cells from dividing too quickly. When the genes (brakes) don't work correctly, cells begin to grow out of control, which can lead to cancer. Many different tumor suppressor genes have been identified, including the BRCA1, BRCA2, APC, p53, and RB1 genes.[9]

Cancer develops over time as an accumulation of many molecular changes. An astronomically large number of cell divisions have to occur during the process. Human tumors usually do not become apparent until they have grown to a size of 10–100 billion cells. It normally takes decades to accumulate enough mutations to produce a tumor that can be diagnosed as malignant.[10]

Cancer incidence increases with age. Exposure to carcinogens increases the likelihood that harmful changes will occur, and increases the probability of developing cancer during a normal life span. If a person has inherited a cancer-susceptibility mutation and it is in all of the body's cells from birth, then that accumulation of changes may take place in a much shorter time frame.[11]

Thinking about the development of cancer as a multi-step process can help explain the lag time that often separates exposure to a cancer-causing agent and the development of cancer, such as severe childhood sunburns that develop into skin cancer years later. It can also explain the 20– to 25–year lag between the onset of widespread cigarette smoking among women after World War II and the massive increase in lung cancer that occurred among women in the 1970s.[12]

There are about 200 different types of cancer, each one classified by the type of cell that is initially affected.[13]

Normal cells in the body follow an orderly path of growth, division, and death. Unlike regular cells, cancer cells do not experience programmed death, but instead continue to grow and divide. This leads to a mass of abnormal cells that grow out of control.[14]

Cancer proceeds through three stages: initiation, promotion, and progression.[15] The DNA damage can take place in a matter of hours or even minutes, and is considered the first stage of possible cancer.

1st Stage Minutes/Hours	2nd Stage Years/Decades	3rd Stage After Diagnosis
Initiation DNA Damage	Promotion	Progression and Metastasis

One cell may become cancerous and begin to divide. The average doubling time is about 3.5 months. After 6 years, you could have a cancer growth the size of the tip of a lead pencil, which is undetectable by any test we have. If it is aggressive, it has metastasized (spread) to other parts of the body, still without being detected.[16]

On average, at about 10 years of growth, the cancer becomes a tumor mass the size of a pencil eraser. Depending upon where it is located, it may be felt at this time. Mammograms usually don't pick up breast cancer until it has been growing nearly 14 years. The promotion (second) stage of cancer growth is during the 10–20 years it grows undetected in your body.[17]

During the third stage (progression) of this multi-step cancer growth, the advanced cancer cells begin to invade and are considered malignant. In the final stage, the tumor actually breaks away and starts wandering, or metastasizing. This eventually results in death.[18]

As you can see, cancer doesn't "just happen" the month before the diagnosis. Even though the tumor may have been growing for years, the day you go into the doctor's office and get the results of your tests is the day you become "sick." From this explanation, you can see the fallacy of what we like to call "early detection."

Chapter 3:
Cancer Risk Factors by Type of Cancer

*Cancer is a word,
not a sentence.*

~ John Diamond

W e hear about some new form of environmental risk that is linked to cancer on a regular basis and we worry about each one for the moment, but eventually it becomes overwhelming. I have organized this chapter by type of some of the most common cancers and the risk factors that go with each one. You can read about all of them, or you can just peek at the ones you're most interested in.

Bladder Cancer

Bladder cancer is more common in industrialized countries such as the United States, Canada, and France. Its incidence is lowest in Asia and South America. It occurs more frequently in men than in women, and in people of lower socioeconomic status.[1]

The most important risk factor for developing bladder cancer is cigarette smoking and other tobacco use; other risk factors include occupational exposure in the dye, leather, or rubber industries. Certain parasitic infections, such as schistosomiasis, are associated with a high incidence of bladder cancer.[2] You get a schistosoma infection through contact with contaminated water. It is not usually seen in the United States, but this infection is common in many tropical areas worldwide.[3]

A recent study found that those who ate the most red meat, especially when it's well-done or cooked at high temperatures, were almost 1.5 times more likely to develop bladder cancer than those who ate the least. According to study author Dr. Xifeng Wu, "These results strongly support what we suspected: people who eat a lot of red meat, particularly well-done red meat, such as fried or barbecued, seem to have a higher likelihood of bladder cancer."[4]

Other possible risk factors include heavy coffee consumption, treatment with chlornaphazine or cyclophosphamide (anti-cancer drugs), long-term use of pain killers containing phenacetin (a chemical which was removed from medications and hair dyes in 1983), urinary tract infections, low urine flow, or genetic factors.[5]

Convincing evidence also points to egg consumption as a source of increased risk for bladder cancer. A case-control study of 130 newly diagnosed bladder cancer patients, published in the journal *International Urology and Nephrology*, determined that moderate egg consumption tripled the risk of developing bladder cancer.[6] In Uruguay, people with bladder cancer were studied, and it was found that consumption of barbecued meat, salted meat, and fried eggs "were associated with significant increased risks of bladder cancer."[7]

Brain Cancer

The cause of primary brain tumors is unknown. This is because they are rare, there are many types, and there are many possible risk factors that could play a role. Exposure to some types of radiation, head injuries, and hormone replacement therapy may be risk factors.[8]

Chemists, embalmers, and workers in the oil refinery and rubber industries show higher rates of brain cancer. Other possible risk factors are exposure to electromagnetic fields, exposure to farm animals and pets, severe head trauma, loud noise, cigarettes, alcohol, and N-nitroso compounds in the diet.[9]

N-nitroso compounds, including N-nitrosodimethyla-mine (NDMA), have been shown to be potent carcinogens in animal experiments. They are found in foods which contain nitrite or have been exposed to nitrogen oxides. Among these are cured meats, especially cooked bacon and Japanese smoked and cured fish. Some German beers are another source of NDMA.[10]

In a report released in August 2009, L. Lloyd Morgan (an electronics engineer, a member of the Bioelectromagnetics Society, and the report's lead author) says, "Exposure to cell phone radiation is the largest human health experiment ever undertaken, without informed consent, and has some 4 billion participants enrolled. Science has shown increased risk of brain tumors from use of cell phones, as well as increased risk of eye cancer, salivary gland tumors, testicular cancer, non-Hodgkin's lymphoma, and leukemia. The public must be informed."[11]

Tumors may occur at any age, but many specific tumors have a particular age group in which they are most common. In adults, gliomas and meningiomas are the most common types of brain tumors.[12] Meningiomas are a generally curable kind of brain cancer, while gliomas are more life-threatening.

A 2004 case-control study suggested an association between hypertension and glioma. The authors hypothesized that this association was mediated through potentially neurocarcinogenic effects of antihypertensive medication.[13]

One especially frightening study found that children who did not eat any fruit in the first year of life had a 430 percent increased risk of developing a brain cancer.[14]

Breast Cancer

One out of eight American women will be diagnosed with this disease during their lifetime—one of the highest rates in the world. This cancer is more common in Caucasians than in other racial groups, although rates have been rising among blacks, Hispanics, and women of Asian origin.[15]

There is overwhelming evidence that estrogen levels are a critical determinant of breast cancer risk.[16] Other risk factors include childlessness, first child born after age 30, high doses of ionizing radiation, long-term use of post-menopause estrogens and progestins, obesity, use of tobacco products, excessive alcohol consumption, and stress.[17]

Family history (especially in a mother or sister) of breast cancer; personal history of breast, ovarian, or endometrial cancer; susceptibility genes (BRCA-1, BRCA-2); and some forms of benign breast disease (atypical hyperplasia) are also risk factors.[18] However, one research group found that less than 3% of all breast cancer cases can be attributed to family history.[19]

An increase in fish intake has also been associated with an increase in breast cancer. In a study published in the *Journal of Nutrition*, researchers found that for each ounce of lean fish consumed daily there was a 13% increase in risk of breast cancer.[20]

Women with higher levels of insulin-like growth factor 1 (IGF-1) in their blood have a greater risk of premenopausal breast cancer.[21] The Harvard Nurses' Health Study found that women with higher IGF-1 levels had more than double the risk compared to women with lower IGF-1 levels.[22]

We occasionally hear of the reputed benefits of moderate alcohol consumption for reducing heart disease risk, but even one drink per day, if consumed every day, increases breast cancer risk.[23]

Cervical Cancer

Several risk factors increase your chance of developing cervical cancer. Women without any of these risk factors rarely develop the disease.[24]

Risk factors for cervical cancer are infection with human papillomavirus (HPV), early age at first sexual intercourse, many sexual partners or partners who have had many sexual partners, multiple births, long-term oral contraceptive use, and cigarette smoking. Others include family history, obesity, HIV, chlamydia infection, and diethylstilbestrol (DES), a hormonal drug given to women to prevent miscarriage.[25]

Women with very low vitamin C intake can have a cervical cancer risk which is ten times higher than women who consume more dietary vitamin C.[26] Vitamin C intake from fruits and vegetables is a powerful antioxidant.

Colorectal Cancer

Risk factors for colorectal cancer include personal or family history of colorectal polyps or inflammatory bowel disease, certain rare hereditary conditions, a high-fat diet, and a diet low in fiber, fruits or vegetables. Possible risk factors include physical inactivity, alcohol consumption, obesity, and smoking.[27]

In a paper published almost 30 years ago, researchers compared environmental factors and cancer rates in 32 countries around the world. One of the strongest links between any cancer and any dietary factor was between colon cancer and meat intake. The countries where more meat, more animal protein, more sugar, and fewer cereal grains were consumed had far higher rates of colon cancer.[28]

A six-year study of 88,000 nurses by Boston's Brigham and Women's Hospital found that lower red meat intake is associated with lower colon cancer risk; and weight gain is associated with increased risks of colorectal cancer.[29]

There has been some recent press about the value of calcium in treating colon cancer. Unfortunately, that has not been totally proven. In rural China, where calcium consumption is modest and almost no dairy products are consumed, colon cancer rates are much lower than they are in Europe and North America where calcium consumption is high.[30]

A study recently published in the *American Journal of Clinical Nutrition* concluded that, "A family diet rich in dairy products during childhood is associated with a greater risk of colorectal cancer in adulthood."[31]

Another study showed that increased alcohol consumption was a risk factor for liver and colorectal cancer.[32]

In a study of 1,009 colon cancer patients, researchers found that survival depended to a great extent on dietary habits. Those who consumed more red and processed meats, sweets, and refined grains were more likely to have a recurrence of or die from the disease after a median five-year follow-up.[33]

Some very convincing evidence points to egg consumption as a source of increased risk for colorectal cancer. The World Health Organization analyzed data from 34 countries and determined that egg consumption was definitely correlated with mortality from colon and rectal cancers in both men and women.[34]

In Argentina, a study found that people who consumed 1.5 eggs per week had nearly five times more colorectal cancer risk than individuals who consumed fewer than 11 eggs per year.[35]

Endometrial Cancer

Endometrial cancer is the most common form of uterine cancer.[36] It tends to be more common in the United States than in other parts of the world, and it is more frequently found in Caucasian women of higher socioeconomic status.[37]

High cumulative exposure to estrogens include childlessness, bearing few children, beginning menstruation at an early age, failure to menstruate, late menopause, and estrogen replacement therapy are major risk factors. Infertility, use of tamoxifen, obesity, diabetes, hypertension, gallbladder disease, and Stein-Leventhal syndrome (polycystic ovary disease) are other known risk factors.[38]

A study published in the *International Journal of Cancer* provides evidence that animal-derived foods increase the risk of endometrial cancer, while foods from plant sources reduce it. Dr. Wang-Hong Xu and colleagues found that women who received most of their calories from animal protein had twice the risk of developing the disease compared to those who took in the fewest calories from animal sources. Women who ate the most protein from plant sources cut their endometrial cancer risk by 30 percent.[39]

Esophageal Cancer

The most important risk factors for cancer of the esophagus are tobacco use (cigarettes, cigars, and pipes), excessive alcohol use, and Barrett's esophagus (also known as Barrett's syndrome), a condition associated with a long history of gastroesophageal reflux disease (GERD). Other risk factors are obesity, insufficient consumption of fruits and vegetables, high intake of pickles or pickled vegetables, moldy foods, and the consumption of very hot foods and beverages.[40]

People who eat plenty of fruits and vegetables have lower rates of cancer arising in the esophagus.[41]

Gallbladder Cancer

The most important risk factor for gallbladder cancer is gallstones; factors related to stone formation are increasing age, being female, being pregnant, obesity, and the use of estrogen-containing drugs.[42] Another risk factor is porcelain gallbladder (a condition in which the wall of the gallbladder becomes covered with calcium deposits). People chronically infected with salmonella (the bacterium that causes typhoid) and those who are carriers of the disease are more likely to develop gallbladder cancer than those not infected. Risk of gallbladder cancer is highest among Mexican Americans and Native Americans.[43]

Kidney Cancer

Cigarette smoking is the most important risk factor for kidney cancer; others are obesity, occupational exposure to arsenic, and abuse of analgesics, especially pain relievers containing phenacetin. (In the U.S., phenacetin was removed from medications and hair dyes in 1983.) Other risk factors include regular use of prescription diuretics and increased meat consumption.[44]

Laryngeal Cancer

Smokers are far more likely than nonsmokers to get cancer of the larynx. People who drink alcohol are more likely to develop laryngeal cancer than people who don't drink. The risk increases if the person drinks alcohol and also smokes tobacco.[45]

Other risk factors include gastroesophageal reflux disease (GERD), which causes stomach acid to flow up into the esophagus;[46] and occupational exposure to asbestos, sulfuric acid mist, nickel, or mustard gas.[47]

Leukemia

Blood cancers such as leukemia, myeloma, and myelodysplastic syndrome are cancers that originate in the bone marrow. They are considered to be related cancers.[48]

Risk factors include family history of blood cancers; high doses of ionizing radiation; alkylating drugs used in cancer treatments; human T-cell leukemia-lymphoma virus (HTLV-1); Down syndrome or other genetic abnormalities; and occupational exposure to benzene. Other possible risk factors are exposure to electromagnetic fields, pesticides and smoking.[49]

Exposure to high doses of radiation causes leukemia by inducing DNA damage. The association between radiation exposure and leukemia was noted in survivors of the atomic bomb in Japan and in people who lived near the nuclear reactors in the Chernobyl disaster of 1986. Leukemia caused by radiation typically appears 10 years after exposure.[50]

We know that unborn babies exposed to radiation during pelvimetry (X-rays to determine the mother's pelvic size) have a considerably higher incidence of leukemia compared to babies not irradiated while in the uterus.[51]

In 1946, a statistical study of obituaries in the *New England Journal of Medicine* by Dr. Helmuth Ulrich found the leukemia rate among radiologists to be eight times that of other doctors. In 1963, a study by Dr. E. B. Lewis found a significant excess of deaths from leukemia, multiple myeloma, and aplastic anemia among radiologists.[52]

Chemotherapy, which is used for the treatment of other cancers, can cause DNA damage and may increase the risk of developing some form of leukemia. For example, chemotherapy for the treatment of other cancers is the major recognized cause of acute myeloid leukemia in the young, referred to by clinicians as secondary or treatment-related AML.[53]

Cigarette smoke and gasoline contain benzene, another chemical which causes leukemia. Although smoking in the young is associated with modest increases in the risk of developing leukemia, smokers over age 60 may have a twofold increase in risk for AML and a threefold increase in risk for acute lymphoid leukemia (ALL).[54]

The risk of developing leukemia is 10–20 times higher for children with Down syndrome than the general population.[55]

Studies have shown a statistically significant increase in the incidence of ALL in people who live in areas where the cattle have a high incidence of infection.[56]

According to a study published in 2009 in the British Journal of Cancer, cancers of the blood were drastically reduced for vegetarians. Researchers followed 61,000 meat-eaters and vegetarians for over 12 years and found that cancers of the blood were reduced by as much as 45 percent for those following a vegetarian diet. [57]

Liver Cancer

Liver cancer is strongly associated with increasing blood cholesterol. Individuals who are chronically infected with the hepatitis B virus (HBV) and who consume animal-based foods have high blood cholesterol and a higher rate of liver cancer.[58]

Epidemiological studies have shown that obese people have about a 150% increase in their risk of cancer overall and a 450% greater risk of developing liver cancer.[59]

Other risk factors are chronic infection with the

hepatitis C virus, cirrhosis of the liver (chronic liver injury, usually due to alcohol abuse), and occupational exposure to thorium dioxide or vinyl chloride.[60]

Another common health concern is the fear that aflatoxin, which is produced by a mold that grows on peanuts, corn and other grains, causes liver cancer. However, evidence found in *The China Study* strongly indicates that chronic infection with the hepatitis B virus and high serum cholesterol levels are the primary culprits of liver cancer.[61]

According to Dr. Campbell, author of *The China Study*, "We did not find any relationship between aflatoxin and liver cancer, and we have the largest study on this question ever done."[62]

Lung Cancer

Cigarette smoking causes lung cancer. In fact, smoking tobacco is the major risk factor for lung cancer. In the United States, about 90% of lung cancer deaths in men and almost 80% of lung cancer deaths in women are due to smoking. People who smoke are 10–20 times more likely to get lung cancer or die from lung cancer than people who do not smoke.[63]

Secondhand smoke and using cigars or pipes increases the risk for lung cancer.[64]

Radon gas causes lung cancer and is sometimes found in people's homes. Radon is an odorless, colorless gas that comes from rocks and dirt, and it can get trapped in houses and buildings. According to EPA estimates, radon is the number one cause of lung cancer among nonsmokers.[65]

Other risk factors for lung cancer include substances

found at some workplaces, such as asbestos, arsenic, and some forms of silica and chromium. For many of these substances, the risk of getting lung cancer is even higher for those who also smoke.[66]

Lymphomas

Hodgkin's lymphoma, formerly known as Hodgkin's disease, is one of two types of cancers of the lymphatic system. The other type, non-Hodgkin's lymphoma, is much more common.[67]

People who have had infectious mononucleosis (an infection caused by the Epstein-Barr virus) have an increased risk of Hodgkin's disease. Hodgkin's disease is most common in early adulthood (especially in a person's 20s) and in late adulthood (after age 55). Possible risk factors include a family history of Hodgkin's lymphoma, especially among siblings.[68]

"Chronic inflammatory conditions such as rheumatoid arthritis have been associated with malignant lymphomas," explained Dr. Eva Baecklund and colleagues in a study published in *Arthritis and Rheumatism*.[69]

Rheumatoid arthritis (RA) is a disease that occurs when a person's own immune system begins to attack cells around the joints. Lymphoma, on the other hand, is a type of cancer that affects the lymph nodes. The American Cancer Society estimates that over 65,000 people will be diagnosed this year with some type of lymphoma, but those with RA seem to be about twice as likely as the general population to develop this disease, said Dr. John Patrick Whelan, pediatric rheumatologist at Massachusetts

General Hospital for Children.[70]

In Norway, a large study followed almost 16,000 individuals for more than 11 years and found a strong positive association between lymphoma and milk. If a person drank two or more glasses of milk daily, the odds of developing lymphoma were 3.4 times greater than persons drinking less than one glass of milk.[71]

Most people with non-Hodgkin's lymphoma are older than 60. Researchers are studying obesity and other possible risk factors for non-Hodgkin's lymphoma. People who work with herbicides or certain other chemicals may be at increased risk of this disease. Researchers are also looking at a possible link between using hair dyes before 1980 and non-Hodgkin's lymphoma.[72]

Infections such as HIV, Epstein-Barr, Helicobacter pylori (*H. pylori*), and hepatitis C can increase the risk of lymphoma.[73]

Some research findings show that increased exposure to sunshine improves survival for people who already have cancer, including those with lymphoma.[74]

Melanoma

Risk factors are excessive exposure to ultraviolet radiation (sunlight), fair skin, history of severe sunburns, personal or family history of melanoma, multiple or atypical moles (colored skin spots), giant congenital moles, personal history of melanoma, and reduced immune function due to organ transplants or HIV infection. Melanoma occurs almost exclusively among Caucasians.[75]

In a report issued by the World Health Organization,

ultraviolet radiation tanning beds and UV radiation were moved up to the highest cancer risk category. Dr. Fatiha El Ghissassi and colleagues at IARC in Lyon, France, conducted a comprehensive meta-analysis and concluded that the risk of skin melanoma is increased by 75% when the use of tanning devices starts before 30 years of age.[76]

The risk for developing melanoma is directly related to the degree to which the immune system is suppressed. For example, individuals who have undergone organ transplants and are taking anti-rejection medication have 3 times the risk of developing melanoma, basal cell, or squamous cell cancers of the skin.[77]

The most serious warning about melanoma is to stay out of the sun, but some conflicting research shows that sun exposure has little to do with the cause of melanoma. There is good evidence that sunshine can help prevent this cancer, and even slow its growth. Melanoma is believed to be due to a diet low in fruits and vegetables and high in fats and vegetable oils.[78]

Oral Cancer

Tobacco and alcohol usage account for most mouth cancers. Another risk factor is a diet low in fruits and vegetables. Other possible risk factors include poor tooth development and oral hygiene, trauma due to ill-fitting dentures or jagged teeth, use of mouthwashes with high alcohol content, and iron-deficiency anemia.[79]

Mouth cancer can occur in any part of the mouth, tongue, lips, throat, salivary glands, pharynx, larynx, sinuses, and other areas of the head and neck. Heavy drinkers who smoke are 30 times more likely to get the disease. Early detection of the disease increases survival chances from just 50% to 90%.[80]

A high proportion of oropharyngeal cancers in non-smokers and younger adults have been associated with human papillomavirus (HPV). The mode of transmission may be frequent oral sex in adolescents and young adults.[81] According to a report in the *British Medical Journal*, "four or more oral sex partners in a lifetime are all a person needs to up their risk of contracting a cancer-causing strain of HPV."[82]

Ovarian Cancer

Risk factors are personal history of breast cancer, family history of breast or ovarian cancer, susceptibility genes (BRCA-1, BRCA-2), childlessness, and hereditary non-polyposis colon cancer. A possible risk factor is dietary fat. Risk may be reduced by hysterectomy and tubal ligation.[83]

Ovarian cancer is more common in the United States than in Asian countries, and it occurs more frequently in countries where breast, colon, and endometrial cancers tend to occur. It tends to be more common in higher socio-economic groups and less frequent in women who use oral contraceptives.[84]

Researchers at Johns Hopkins University found that the higher a woman's cholesterol level—which reflects a fattier diet—the greater her risk of developing ovarian cancer.[85]

There is some evidence that indicates milk may increase the risk of ovarian cancer. Dr. Daniel Cramer of Harvard

University compared the diets of hundreds of women with ovarian cancer to a group of women who were similar in age and other demographic variables, but who did not have cancer. He found that the women with ovarian cancer consumed noticeably more dairy products.[86]

Dr. Cramer's concern was the milk sugar, which is also called lactose. Lactose is made of two smaller sugars called glucose and galactose. Galactose is potentially toxic to the ovaries and is linked with higher rates of infertility.[87]

Enzymes usually help the body eliminate galactose, but some women have particularly low levels of these enzymes. When these women consume dairy products regularly, their risk of ovarian cancer is triple that of other women.[88]

Galactose is present in all milk products, including yogurt, ice cream, and cheeses—the whole-milk as well as the low-fat varieties.[89]

A recent analysis of studies found that, for every 10 grams of lactose consumed (the amount in one glass of milk), ovarian cancer risk increased by 13%.[90]

Consumption of eggs was associated with an increased risk of ovarian cancer in a study of 29,083 postmenopausal women done at the University of Minnesota.[91]

Pancreatic Cancer

Although the exact causes of pancreatic cancer are unknown, several risk factors appear to be linked with the disease:

> ⩔ Age: The likelihood of developing pancreatic cancer increases with age, with most people being over the age of 60 when the cancer is diagnosed.

- ☙ Race: In the U.S., African-Americans are more likely to develop pancreatic cancer than Caucasians or Asian-Americans.

- ☙ Smoking: Cigarette smokers are 2 to 3 times more likely than nonsmokers to develop pancreatic cancer, and about 3 out of every 10 cases of pancreatic cancer are found to be linked to smoking. Cigarettes, cigars, and chewing tobacco all increase pancreatic cancer risk. Cigarette smoke contains chemicals called nitrosamines, which are carcinogenic.

- ☙ Diet: A diet high in meat and fat increases the risk of pancreatic cancer, whereas eating more fruits and vegetables appears to offer some protection. A diet high in folate (folic acid) has been shown to reduce the risk of pancreatic cancer, but folate supplements have not been shown to reduce the risk. Folate is found in leafy, green vegetables.

- ☙ Diabetes: Pancreatic cancer is more common in people with diabetes.

- ☙ Family history: The risk for developing pancreatic cancer is three times greater if an immediate family member (mother, father, sister, brother) has had the disease.[92]

- ☙ Medical factors: Pancreatic cancer is more common in patients who have a history of cirrhosis, chronic pancreatitis, or surgery to the upper digestive tract.

> ❧ Environmental factors: Pancreatic cancer can result from long-term exposure to certain chemicals, such as gasoline or certain insecticides.[93]

People who drink at least two sugary sodas a week have an increased risk of developing cancer of the pancreas; and a recent study shows that researchers suspect the culprit is sugar. The data analyzed for the soda study came from the Singapore Chinese Health Study, which enrolled more than 63,000 Singaporeans who lived in government housing estates—as nearly 9 in 10 people in Singapore do—and looked at their diets, physical activity, and medical history.[94]

"A typical serving of soda is 20 ounces and contains 65 grams of sugar. By comparison, a typical serving of orange juice is 8 ounces and contains 21 grams of sugar," said Mark Pereira of the University of Minnesota's Division of Epidemiology and Community Health, who is one of the authors of the study.[95]

In a study published in the *Journal of the American Medical Association*, scientists found that people who took on excess weight in early adulthood or even their teens are at greatest risk for pancreatic cancer. Obesity and smoking are the major modifiable risk factors associated with the disease. About 25% of pancreatic cancer cases are associated with obesity and 27% with smoking.[96]

Prostate Cancer

High prostate cancer rates primarily exist in societies with Western diets and lifestyles.[97] In a 2001 Harvard review of the research, it was found that men with the highest dairy intakes had approximately double the risk of total prostate cancer.[98]

In another review of published literature done in 1998, the conclusion was that meats, dairy products, and eggs were frequently associated with a higher risk of prostate cancer.[99] Men with higher than normal blood levels of IGF-1 have been shown to have 5.1 times the risk of advanced-stage prostate cancer.[100] An enormous body of evidence shows that animal products are associated with prostate cancer.[101]

Other studies have shown that infertile men have an increased risk of developing an aggressive form of prostate cancer which may warrant early screening.[102]

Stomach Cancer

Risk factors for stomach cancer are dietary nitrites (found in pickled, salted, and smoked foods), pernicious anemia, and diets low in fruits and vegetables. Possible risk factors are infection with *H. pylori*, high doses of ionizing radiation, cigarette smoking, and genetic factors.[103]

Gastric adenocarcinoma (stomach cancer) is the second leading cause of cancer death worldwide. It has been suggested that consumption of salty foods causes this cancer, but current research does not support this belief.[104] Consumption of red and processed meat, along with the lack of fruits and vegetables, have been documented to be major causes of this deadly cancer.[105]

One study conducted by researchers from NCI's Division of Cancer Epidemiology and Genetics found a link between individuals with stomach cancer and the consumption of cooked meats. The researchers assessed the diets and cooking habits of 176 people diagnosed with stomach cancer and 503 people without cancer. The researchers found that those who ate their beef medium well or well done had more than three times the risk of stomach cancer than those who ate their beef rare or medium rare. They also found that people who ate beef four or more times a week had more than twice the risk of stomach cancer than those consuming beef less often.[106]

Another possible risk factor may be tied to increases in lower esophageal cancers caused by gastric reflux from abdominal obesity.[107]

Thyroid Cancer

Risk factors for thyroid cancer are high doses of ionizing radiation and goiter.[108] Possible risk factors which are still being studied include soy and soy products. Goiter and hypothyroidism have been reported in infants receiving soy formula. Autoimmune diseases of the thyroid and thyroid cancer may also be caused by exposure to soy.[109]

A recent study done in Kuwait suggests that low-dose diagnostic radiation exposure may be associated with the risk of thyroid cancer. The study abstract stated, "An increased risk of thyroid cancer has been reported in dentists, dental assistants, and x-ray workers."[110]

Chapter 4:
Cancer Risk Factors
by Type of Hazard

*A recipe for early death is to just
eat whatever you want*

~ John Mackey

Scientists estimate that as many as 50%–75% of cancer deaths in the United States are caused by human behaviors such as smoking, physical inactivity, and poor dietary choices.[1] According to the best assessments of the National Cancer Institute, 80%–90% of cancers are attributable to environmental factors. Within those environmental factors, 30% of cancers are caused by tobacco and even more cases—from 30% to 60%—are caused by foods.[2]

As previously discussed, cancers are usually caused by many factors. A carcinogen is something that can help to cause cancer. Tobacco smoke is a powerful carcinogen. But not everyone who smokes gets lung cancer. So there must be other factors at work as well as carcinogens.

Cancer can start in any type of body tissue. What affects one body tissue may not affect another. For example, tobacco smoke that you breathe in may help to cause lung cancer. Overexposing your skin to the sun could cause a melanoma on your leg. But the sun won't give you lung cancer, and smoking won't necessarily give you melanoma.[3]

Numerous risk factors have been shown to genetically transform normal cell DNA into cancer-prone cells. Even though you may have many of these cancer-prone cells, they will not grow and multiply until the right conditions are in place. That is why it is so important to minimize your risks in the first place to prevent the mutations; by keeping your risk factors low, you will also be able to thwart many of those cancer-prone cells from multiplying and growing.

The risk of developing cancer increases as we age, so

age—along with gender, race, and personal and family medical history—is a risk factor for cancer.[4] Other risk factors besides lifestyle choices include certain infections, occupational exposures, and some environmental factors.

John Mackey, CEO of the Whole Foods grocery chain, lists the top six risk factors or causes of cancer in order of importance:

- Diet (30%–60%)
- Tobacco (30%)
- Pollution (5%)
- Alcohol (3%)
- Radiation (3%)
- Medication (2%)[5]

If you were to think about everything you have ever read or heard about the causes of cancer, I bet you would be able to make a very long list. In this chapter, I am going to list some of the major and minor risk factors of cancer. For simplicity's sake, I have elected to list them alphabetically.

Age

Most types of cancer become more common as we get older. This is because the changes that make a cell become cancerous in the first place take a long time to develop. The longer we live, the more time we have for genetic mistakes to happen in our cells.

The repair of damaged DNA is critical to our survival.

While free radicals continuously bombard our DNA, our repair enzymes correct about 98% of the damage.[6] The better we can protect our DNA using foods containing antioxidants, the lower our risk of developing cancer.[7]

As we age, our cell repair process becomes less and less efficient. This helps explain why cancer is significantly more common after age 65.[8]

Alcohol

The association of alcohol consumption with increased risk for breast cancer has been a consistent finding in a majority of epidemiologic studies during the past two decades. Alcoholic beverages raise estrogen and andro-gen levels in women and, as a consequence, may increase the risk of breast cancer.[9] A study reported in the *Journal of the American Medical Association* found that alcoholic drinks tripled blood estrogen levels among women under-going estrogen-replacement therapy.[10]

Drinking a lot of alcohol has also been shown to increase a person's chance of getting cancer of the mouth, larynx, esophagus, breast, and liver. This is especially true if the alcohol drinker also smokes.[11]

Women who consumed three or more alcoholic drinks a day increased their breast cancer risk by more than 50% compared to nondrinkers.[12] People who drink alcohol should limit their intake to no more than two drinks per day for men and one drink per day for women. A drink is defined as 12 ounces of beer, 5 ounces of wine, or 1.5 ounces of 80-proof distilled spirits. Women at high risk of breast cancer may want to consider not drinking any alcohol.[13]

Acrylamide

Acrylamide is a chemical produced industrially for use in products such as plastics and cosmetics. Cigarette smoke is another major source of exposure to acrylamide. The chemical is considered to be a probable human carcinogen, based mainly on studies in laboratory animals.[14]

It has also been found in certain foods made from plants, such as potato products, grain products, or coffee.[15] Especially high levels have been found in potato chips and french fries.[16]

Food storage and preparation methods to lower acrylamide levels include:

> Roasting (rather than frying) potato pieces causes less acrylamide formation, followed by baking whole potatoes. Boiling potatoes and microwaving whole potatoes with skin does not produce acrylamide.

> Soaking raw potato slices in water for 15–30 minutes before frying or roasting helps reduce acrylamide formation during cooking.

> Storing potatoes in the refrigerator can result in increased acrylamide during cooking. Therefore, store potatoes outside the refrigerator; preferably in a dark, cool place, such as a closet or a pantry, to prevent sprouting.

> Generally, more acrylamide accumulates when

food is cooked for longer periods or at higher temperatures. Cooking cut potato products, such as frozen french fries or potato slices, to a golden yellow color rather than a brown color helps reduce acrylamide formation. Brown areas tend to contain more acrylamide.

> Toasting bread to a light brown color, rather than a dark brown color, lowers the amount of acrylamide. Very brown areas should be avoided, since they contain the most acrylamide.

> Acrylamide forms in coffee when coffee beans are roasted, not when coffee is brewed at home or in a restaurant. So far, scientists have not found good ways to reduce acrylamide formation in coffee.[17]

> Steam or boil potatoes and green and yellow vegetables.

> When baking breads or casseroles, using lower temperatures for longer periods of time will produce less acrylamide.

> Removing the crust from commercial breads will also reduce acrylamide exposure.[18]

Arachidonic Acid

A significant number of studies have linked diets high in arachidonic acid to tumor growth and increased inflammation. Some foods which contain high levels of arachidonic acid include:

> Almonds

> Chicken

> Coconut

> Egg yolk

> Hazelnuts

> Macadamia nuts

> Peanuts

> Pecans

> Pistachios

> Red meat

> Walnuts

> Whole-milk dairy products[19]

Chronic Disease

People suffering from certain chronic inflammatory diseases such as rheumatoid arthritis, lupus, or a parasitic infection seem to have a higher risk for cancer than the general public. People infected with the hepatitis B or C viruses have a higher incidence of liver cancer than uninfected people.[20]

Cholesterol

High cholesterol levels, a risk factor that we know is associated with heart disease, has also been correlated with many cancers.[21]

Total cholesterol levels of less than 200 mg/dL are considered desirable for Americans as published in guidelines by the American Heart Association.[22] The average blood cholesterol of Americans is 215 mg/dL, while the average for the Chinese is only 127 mg/dL.[23]

One important finding from research done during the China project was that, as blood cholesterol levels in rural China *decreased* from 170 mg/dL to 90 mg/dL, cancers of the liver, rectum, colon, lung, breast, bone marrow, brain, stomach, and esophagus (throat) also decreased.[24]

If blood cholesterol is an important indicator of disease, how can we lower our risk? Animal-based foods are corre-lated with increasing blood cholesterol, while plant-based foods are associated with decreasing blood cholesterol.[25]

What is the difference between fat and cholesterol? Fat is visible as a yellow layer under a chicken skin or white streaks marbled through a cut of beef. Cholesterol, on the other hand, resides as tiny particles inside the cell within an animal's body, primarily in the lean portion.[26] Because fish and chicken are animals, they have just as much cho-lesterol as beef or pork.[27]

Your liver makes all the cholesterol your body needs for normal function, so there is no need for any choles-terol in your diet.[28]

Dairy Products

Most dairy products (milk, cheese, yogurt, ice cream, etc.) are loaded with fat and cholesterol, and research-ers are discovering that dairy products appear to play an important role in cancer risk. Harvard researchers in the Physicians' Health Study and the Health Professionals

Follow-Up Study found that men who frequently consumed dairy products had a higher prostate cancer risk.[29]

Milk is high in fat and has no fiber at all. In addition, milk appears to interfere with the activation of vitamin D in the body. Vitamin D is actually a hormone that helps your body absorb calcium from the digestive tract and helps to protect against prostate cancer.[30]

Other possible reasons for this connection include the tendency of dairy products to boost IGF-1 production in the body; and the high calcium content of dairy products, which decreases the activation of vitamin D.[31]

According to *The China Study*, the protein which most consistently promoted all stages of the cancer process was casein, which makes up 87% of a cow's milk protein.[32]

Breast cancer and ovarian cancer have also been examined for their links to the consumption of dairy products.[33] In a study done at the University of Illinois Medical Center in Chicago, a research group working with mammary cancer in rats found that increasing intakes of casein promoted the development of mammary cancer.[34]

Dietary Fat

Fatty diets are associated with increased risk of cancer, especially with saturated fat, which is the kind of fat found in meat, dairy products, eggs, and chocolate.[35]

Breast cancer has been associated more with animal fat intake than with plant fat. In *The China Study*, findings showed that reducing total dietary fat from 24% to 6% was associated with lower breast cancer risk.[36]

Fiber

According to studies by the late Professor Denis Burkitt, who traveled across Africa looking at the diets of the African people, people who don't consume enough fiber are susceptible to colon and rectal cancer, diverticulosis, hemorrhoids, and varicose veins.[37]

High fiber intake was consistently associated with lower rates of cancers of the colon and rectum. Beans, leafy vegetables, and whole grains are all high in fiber. Fiber is found only in plant foods such as fruits, vegetables, nuts, and whole grains. Eggs, dairy products, and meats do not contain any form of fiber.[38]

Fluoride

The possible relationship between fluoridated water and cancer has been debated at length. Some studies have shown that fluoride can boost the potency of carcinogens and increase tumor growth by as much as 25%.[39]

In 1990, a study by the National Toxicology Program, which is part of the National Institute of Environmental Health Sciences, showed an increased number of bone tumors in male rats that were given water high in fluoride for two years. However, other studies in humans and in animals have not shown an association between fluoridated water and cancer.[40]

Food Additives

Possible risks have been suggested with aspartame, MSG, hydrolyzed vegetable protein (a form of MSG), soy protein, or the additive carrageenan.

Questions about artificial sweeteners and cancer arose when early studies showed that cyclamate in combination with saccharin caused bladder cancer in laboratory animals. However, results from subsequent carcinogenicity studies (studies that examine whether a substance can cause cancer) on these sweeteners and other approved sweeteners have not provided clear evidence of an association between artificial sweeteners and cancer in people.[41]

Joanne Tobacman, M.D., assistant professor of clinical internal medicine at the University of Iowa and researcher on carrageenan, said, "There seems to be enough evidence associating carrageenan with significant gastrointestinal lesions, including malignancies, to avoid ingesting it."[42]

Carrageenan comes from algae or seaweed and is used as a thickening agent in yogurt, ice cream and chocolate milk. Many sliced deli meats are enriched with carrageenan. In its jelled form, carrageenan is also marketed as a personal lubricant.[43]

Foods We Eat

As researchers have compared the habits and diets of people who developed cancer with those who remained healthy, they have found many factors that influence cancer risk, including certain foods.[44] Many studies have shown that cancer is more common in populations consuming fatty foods and much less common in countries with diets rich in vegetables, fruits, and grains.[45]

The China project found that people who eat the most

animal protein have the most diagnoses of heart disease, cancer, and diabetes. Animal protein consumption in the China project was associated with taller and heavier people, but was also associated with higher levels of total and bad cholesterol. Another finding was that body weight combined with animal protein intake was associated with more cancer.[46]

About one-third of all cancer deaths are related to nutrition, obesity, or physical inactivity. We know that our diet (what we eat) is linked to some types of cancer, but the exact reasons are not yet clear. The best advice is to eat a lot of fresh fruits and vegetables and whole grains.[47]

For many children, chicken nuggets, soft drinks, potato chips, and other assorted forms of junk food are the usual fare. Not only are these children's eating patterns being directed to a lifetime of similar trash foods, but the damage that will eventually lead to cancer is being established at a tender age.[48]

Free Radicals

The free radical theory of aging was conceived by Denham Harman in the 1950s.[49] In later years, the free radical theory was expanded to include not only aging itself, but also age-related diseases. Free radical damage within cells has been linked to a range of disorders; including cancer, arthritis, atherosclerosis, Alzheimer's disease, and diabetes.

Of all free radicals in our bodies, 95% come from our

own metabolism. If we *slow* our metabolism, we produce fewer free radicals. This might explain why animals that are fed low-calorie diets live longer and have fewer cancers: they are producing fewer free radicals. The opposite is also true. If you *increase* your metabolism, you produce more free radicals—a lot more. This may explain why animals on high-calorie diets have more cancers and overall shorter life spans.[50]

When we exercise intensely, our metabolism not only increases dramatically while we are working out, but it remains increased for hours afterward, which means we are producing a storm of free radicals.[51]

Normally, the body can handle free radicals, but if antioxidants are unavailable or if the free radical production becomes excessive, then damage can occur. Of particular importance is that free-radical damage accumulates with age.[52] Antioxidants, as antidotes to free radicals, are found in fresh foods like vegetables and fruits.

Animal-based foods lack antioxidant shields and tend to activate free radical production and cell damage, while plant-based foods, with their abundant antioxidants, tend to prevent such damage.[53]

Low glutathione and low magnesium levels in the tissues have been shown to double the number of free radicals being formed. Foods like spinach, beans, peanuts, and whole grain bread can increase magnesium levels, whereas garlic increases levels of glutathione.[54]

Antioxidants are powerful cancer fighters mainly found in vegetables and fruits. They assist in halting free radical damage, which can otherwise lead to cancer development.[55]

Grapefruit

In a study of 46,000 postmenopausal women published in the *British Journal of Cancer*, it was found that eating grapefruit might actually increase breast cancer risk.[56]

Researchers at the University of Southern California followed these women from 1993 to 2002. Upon analysis, they found that those who ate the most grapefruit had a 30% higher risk of breast cancer than did those who ate no grapefruit.[57]

The investigators noted that estrogen interacts with grapefruit, and that at least two earlier studies found higher levels of estrogen in women who eat a lot of grapefruit or drink a lot of grapefruit juice. This is such a well-known effect that the FDA requires hormone replacement products to carry a label warning that grapefruit juice may increase their potency.[58]

Increased levels of estrogen are the result of consuming diets high in fat and animal protein and low in dietary fiber.[59] That may have been a factor in the grapefruit study.

Genes

Genes play a role in every aspect of our body, from defining traits such as skin and eye color to influencing the development of cancer. Scientists believe that approximately 10% of ovarian epithelial cancer can be attributed to inherited mutations in the BRCA1 and BRCA2 genes.[60] The BRCA genes are tumor suppressor genes—they keep tumors from growing. Mutations in these genes can be inherited from parents. When they are mutated, they no longer suppress abnormal growth, and cancer is more likely to develop.[61]

One research group found that less than 3% of all breast cancer can be attributed to the BRCA genes.[62] So although women with one of these genes are individually more likely to get breast cancer, most breast cancers are not caused by a high-risk, inherited gene fault. The good news is that about half of the women who carry these rare, potent genes do not get cancer.[63]

Hormones

Hormone levels are considered to be risk factors for breast cancer. There are at least four important breast cancer risks:

> Early age of menarche (first menstruation)

> High blood cholesterol

> Late menopause

> High exposure to female hormones[64]

If you eat a diet *high* in animal foods and refined carbohydrates, it will:

> Lower the age of menarche

> Raise the age of menopause

> Increase female hormone levels

> Increase blood cholesterol levels[65]

A study in the *Journal of the National Cancer Institute*

reported that women with naturally high levels of estrogen are four times more likely to develop breast cancer than women who have lower levels of the hormone.[66]

Estrogen-replacement therapy, commonly prescribed for menopausal and postmenopausal women, substantially increases the risk of breast cancer. In addition, estrogen-mimicking compounds found in pesticides and soft plastics are associated with increases in breast cancer risk.[67]

In rural China, the age of a girl's first menstrual period ranges from 15 to 19 years old, with an average age of 17 years. The U.S. average is roughly 11 years![68] Because of the early age of menarche, a woman's body is exposed to higher levels of blood hormones such as estrogen for a much longer period of time. The hormone levels remain high throughout a woman's life if she consumes a diet rich in animal-based food.[69]

This makes it clear that we should not have our children consume diets high in animal-based foods. The first seeds of breast cancer can be sown in young girls who are 8 to 10 years of age.[70]

IGF-1

Insulin-like growth factor 1 (IGF-1) is turning out to be a predictor of cancer, just as high cholesterol is a predictor of heart disease. When the IGF-1 levels increase, it favors the development of cancer.[71]

Tall and big people live shorter life spans. You can raise your IGF-1 by adding milk, synthetic soy products (soy burgers, soy hot dogs, and cheeses), meat, poultry, fish, and shellfish to your diet.[72]

Eating more animal protein enhances the production of this growth hormone (IGF-1) which in turn enhances cancer cell growth. People with higher than normal levels of IGF-1 have been shown to have 5.1 times the risk of advanced-stage prostate cancer. Fundamental to all is the fact that animal-based foods like meat and dairy lead to more IGF-1, which increases cancer risk.[73]

To prevent cancer, you don't want to grow faster or to age faster, and you certainly don't want your disease to grow faster because of increased levels of IGF-1.[74]

Immune System

Some studies have shown that the greatest risk for developing cancer is when cellular immunity falls.[75] Temporary immune deficiencies can develop in the wake of common virus infections; such as influenza, infectious mononucleosis, and measles. Immune responses can also be supressed by blood transfusions, surgery, chemotherapy, malnutrition, smoking, and stress.[76]

People suffering from AIDS-induced immune suppression have a much higher incidence of cancerous tumors, as do people purposefully immunosuppressed for organ transplantation.[77]

Cancer rates dramatically increase with the onset of age-related loss of immune power and continue to increase progressively thereafter.[78]

We know that about 40% of men over the age of 50 have cancer cells in their prostate gland. Yet only a fraction of these men develop full-blown prostate cancer. After the age of 70, the incidence of prostate cancer goes up almost 70%.[79]

The same appears to be true for breast cancers. About 40% of women over the age of 50 have some cancer cells in their breast. Again, however, most will never develop full-blown breast cancer.[80]

It may be that many cancers are not cured, but rather controlled. This would explain the extremely long latent period between the apparent cure of some tumors and their dramatic reappearance many years later. This again emphasizes the importance of keeping your defenses, especially your immune system, in perfect working order.[81]

Studies have shown that vegetarians have approximately double the natural cancer-killer cells of nonvegetarians.[82]

Industrial Pollutants

Considering the fact that several industrial chemicals can cause cancer in people who work with them or in people who live nearby, industrial pollution does not appear to be a major cause of most cancers in the population at large.[83]

Most of us are familiar with the risk factors associated with industrial pollutants, which can include tobacco, ionizing radiation, X-rays, atomic bombs, and above-ground nuclear tests. Cancer-causing chemicals include arsenic, asbestos, and benzene.

Dioxins are chemicals produced through paper and pulp bleaching; burning of municipal, toxic, and hospital wastes; certain electrical fires; and smelters. Dioxins can also be found in some insecticides, herbicides, wood preservatives, and cigarette smoke. There are at least 100 different kinds of dioxins. The most common routes of exposure for dioxins occur through the diet, particularly from animal fats.[84]

Exposure to asbestos (a group of minerals found in housing and industrial building materials) can cause a variety of medical problems, such as mesothelioma.[85]

Studies have shown that people who are exposed to high levels of benzene are at risk for cancer. Benzene is a chemical found in gasoline, cigarette smoke, and other types of pollution.[86]

Pesticides are chemicals used to eliminate or control unwanted or harmful insects, plants, fungi, animals, or microorganisms in order to protect food crops and other plants. Some pesticides have been classified as carcinogens. Chlordane and dichlorodiphenyltrichloroethane (DDT) are possible human carcinogens. General studies of people (such as farmers, pesticide applicators, manufacturers, and crop dusters) with high exposures to pesticides, have found high rates of blood and lymphatic system cancers (leukemias and lymphomas); cancers of the lip, stomach, lung, brain, and prostate; as well as melanoma and other skin cancers.[87]

Fish are also laden with contaminants; of particular concern in recent years are mercury and PCB's. Contamination from these toxins has been linked to increased risks of cancer.[88]

The chemical bisphenol A (BPA), which has been used for years in clear plastic bottles and food can liners, has been restricted in Canada and some U.S. states and municipalities because of potential health effects. Studies have linked it to reproductive abnormalities and a heightened risk of breast and prostate cancers, diabetes, and heart disease.[89]

Even though the evidence isn't conclusive about BPA's link to cancer, Michael Thun, the American Cancer Society's vice president of epidemiology and surveillance research, says limiting exposure is "prudent."[90]

For those who are concerned about BPA exposure, the U.S. National Institute of Environmental Health Sciences recommends these steps:

> Don't microwave polycarbonate plastic food containers. Polycarbonate is strong and durable, but over time it may break down from overuse at high temperatures.

> Polycarbonate containers that contain BPA usually have a #7 on the bottom.

> Reduce your use of canned foods.

> When possible, opt for glass, porcelain or stainless steel containers, particularly for hot food or liquids.

> Use baby bottles that are BPA-free.[91]

Infectious Diseases and Bacteria

Viruses can help cause some cancers, but this does not mean that these cancers can be passed to other people like an infection. It means that the virus can cause genetic changes in cells that make them more likely to become cancerous.[92]

Certain cancers are related to infectious diseases, such as hepatitis B virus (HBV), human papillomavirus (HPV), human immunodeficiency virus (HIV), Helicobacter pylori (*H. pylori*), and others. Many of these could be prevented through behavioral changes, vaccines, or antibiotics.

Practicing unsafe sex can increase your risk of developing HPV, which is a group of over 100 viruses, medically known as human papillomavirus. HPV increases your risk factor for cervical, anal, vulvar, and vaginal cancer.[93]

Cancer is a significant cause of mortality and morbidity in people infected with HIV. The majority of cancers affecting HIV-positive people are those established as AIDS-defining: Kaposi's sarcoma, non-Hodgkin's lymphoma, and invasive cervical cancer.[94]

Epstein-Barr virus (EBV) is very common. People who catch it late in life get glandular fever and have an increased risk of lymphoma. In *The China Study*, EBV infection (together with other unknown factors) contributed to nasopharyngeal cancer.[95]

Bacterial infections have not been traditionally thought of as cancer-causing agents. But recent studies have shown that people who have an *H. pylori* infection in their stomach develop inflammation of the stomach lining, which increases the risk of stomach cancer.[96]

An *H. pylori* infection is thought to be spread through contaminated food and water or through direct mouth-to-mouth contact. In most populations, the bacterium is first acquired during childhood. Some evidence links *H. pylori* to gastric cancer, mucosa-associated lymphoid tissue (MALT), lymphoma, pancreatic cancer and cardiovascular disease.[97]

Inflammation

There is much evidence that chronic inflammation leads to an increased cancer risk. The longer the inflammation persists, the higher the risk of associated cancer.[98]

Dangerous chronic inflammation occurs when the immune system stays turned on and starts attacking healthy cells. Acute (short-term) inflammation is a good thing, as our bodies send cells or agents to deal with an infection or a foreign body, such as a splinter.[99]

Chronic inflammation can be produced by a poor diet, yet numerous nutrients in fruits and vegetables can dramatically reduce inflammation.[100]

Certain types of fats can dramatically increase free radical production by promoting inflammation. A diet high in sweets, especially sweetened soft drinks, can also greatly increase free radical production. Combine this with a typical Western diet devoid of fruits and vegetables, and you have all the makings of a higher risk for cancer.[101]

The C-reactive protein (CRP) test is a blood test that measures chronic inflammation. It is nonspecific—it does not tell you the source of the inflammation, just whether you have it. The inflammation could be coming from an infection in your toe, arthritis in your knuckles, a bad cold, the trauma of a motorcycle accident, or even the active phases of atherosclerosis, which inflames the walls of your arteries.[102]

Chronic inflammation is implicated in all stages of cancer—initiation, promotion, and progression. The body tries to heal itself from the trauma or the unhealthy foods, but it can't overcome the insistence of continued injuries.[103]

Iron and Copper

Excess iron and copper in the body encourages the formation of cancer-causing free radicals.[104] Of course, the body needs a certain amount of iron for healthy blood cells. But beyond this rather small amount, iron becomes a dangerous substance. Because of this, research studies have shown that higher amounts of iron in the blood mean higher cancer risk.[105]

Once iron is absorbed by the digestive tract, the body stores it. Most of us accumulate much more iron than we need. In spite of the advertising from iron supplement manufacturers, "iron overload" is much more common in America than iron deficiency. The reason is the daily diet of red meats and vitamin supplements, which contributes much more iron than most people can safely handle over the long run. A diet of grains, vegetables, fruits, and beans provides adequate iron, without the risk of overload.[106]

Unfortunately, the body has no way to rid itself of excess iron. Believe it or not, the only way to predictably reduce excessive iron stores is by donating blood. So this altruistic act can have health benefits for the donor as well.[107]

Other recommendations are to:

> Avoid almost all multivitamin/multimineral pills because they contain copper and/or iron.

> Avoid eating all kinds of meats because they are plentiful in both minerals. Copper and iron are much more bio-available from meat than from vegetable foods. Liver and shellfish are particularly high in copper. Red meat is

particularly high in bio-available iron.

> Avoid drinking water with elevated copper content. Eighty percent of the homes in the US have copper pipes for water. Check levels in your water. A reverse osmosis device can be installed on the tap used for drinking and cooking water.[108]

Low Vitamin C and Vitamin D Intake

In *The China Study*, it was found that low levels of vitamin C in cancer-prone families increased the incidence of cancer. Cancer rates were five to eight times higher for areas where fruit intake was lowest. Eating fruits clearly showed a powerful antioxidant effect against a variety of diseases.[109]

It has also been found that we need to have an active form of vitamin D (called supercharged D) in our body that we get from food and sunshine (15-30 minutes every couple of days). Our diet can determine how much of this supercharged vitamin is produced. The production of vitamin D in our bodies is not only affected by the foods we eat, but by sunlight, too.[110]

Eating animal protein can *block* the production of supercharged D, leaving the body with low levels of this vitamin D in the blood. Also, if you consume a consistently *high* level of calcium, the levels of supercharged D can decline. Persistently low levels of supercharged D can create an inviting environment for many cancers.[111]

Meat

Scientists in London found that people who consume

a diet high in red meat had significantly higher levels of N-nitroso compounds (which can increase the risk of developing colon cancer) than people who consumed a vegetarian diet.[112]

Carcinogens are sometimes present in foods. For example, when chicken, fish, or red meat is cooked at a high temperature, cancer-causing chemicals called hetero-cyclic amines tend to form. The longer and hotter meat is cooked, the more these compounds form. Grilled chicken has turned out to be largest source of heterocyclic amines in the U.S. diet.[113]

Why should meat contribute to cancer risk? To begin with, its fat content is virtually always much higher than that of plant products. Even skinless chicken breast has a surprising amount of fat. Since meat is not a plant product, it never has any fiber at all. The more you fill up on meat, the less room you have for fiber-rich foods.[114]

Eating red meat increases the chances of dying prema-turely, according to a large federal study that offers power-ful new evidence that a diet that regularly includes steaks, burgers, and pork chops is hazardous to your health.[115]

A study of more than 500,000 middle-aged and elderly Americans found that those who consumed the equiva-lent of about a small hamburger every day were 30% more likely to die, mostly from heart disease and cancer, during the 10 years in which they were followed. Sausage, cold cuts, and other processed meats also increased the risk.[116]

Medication
Medication taken over a long period of time can

seriously deplete the body's nutritional stores. For example, oral contraceptives lower the levels of many nutrients, which can increase the risk for cancer of the cervix, breast, and colon.[117]

Antiseizure medications, blood pressure medications, antiulcer medications, and one type of antidiabetic medication can dramatically lower folate levels. Antihypertensive medications used to control blood pressure also cause loss of nutrients.[118]

It has been shown that women who take drugs that deplete folate, such as the antiseizure medication phenobarbital or phenytoin, have a very high risk of their children developing a nervous system tumor (neuroblastoma) sometime after birth.[119]

Obesity

Obesity is completely preventable.[120]

In the United States, 14% of deaths from cancer in men and 20% of deaths from cancer in women were due to being overweight.[121]

Women who gain weight after age 18 significantly increase their risk of developing breast cancer. Researchers at Harvard University found that women who gained 45 or more pounds were twice as likely to develop cancer, compared with women who gained less than five pounds. The reason may again be related to estrogen. After menopause, most estrogen comes from body fat; the more fat a woman has, the more estrogen she produces.[122]

We're killing our children through bad diets. This is the first generation of children who will not live as long as their parents. We think we're doing our children a favor by giving them treats and their favorite foods, which are filled with sugar, chemicals, and cheese.[123]

The typical American diet consists of:

> Processed foods, oils, sweets, refined grains and pastas, sugars (61%)

> Meat, eggs, dairy, fish (25%)

> Unrefined plant foods (12%; 40% of which is french fries)

> Whole grains (2%)[124]

The average American consumes 28 teaspoons of sugar a day. A 12-ounce soft drink has 10 teaspoons of sugar.[125]

Omega-6 Oils

Several studies have shown that a diet high in the omega-6 fats increases the development and eventual spread of breast cancer in animals. One study, in which the data from 97 different animal studies were analyzed, found that a diet high in the omega-6 fats significantly increased tumor growth. Studies have also shown that obese women with breast cancer, especially those on diets high in the omega-6 fats, had lower survival rates and more advanced disease than thinner women.[126]

A diet high in the omega-6 oils significantly lowers the level of vitamin E in the body, which can then increase the damage by free radicals and can also promote the growth and spread of a tumor. Omega-6 is found in corn, safflower, soybean, sunflower, peanut, and canola oils.[127]

All plants (with a few rare exceptions) contain the

naturally healthy fats known as omega-3 and omega-6 fats in ideal proportions. Simply stay clear of most meat and dairy products and most packaged foods to avoid unhealthy fats.[128]

Polyunsaturated oils derived from vegetables (like corn and safflower oils) are found to be strong promoters of skin cancers in people and experimental animals.[129]

Physical Inactivity

Physical inactivity is strongly linked to prostate, breast, and colorectal cancer. A number of studies have indicated that regular exercise may reduce the risk of breast, colon, and possibly prostate cancers.[130]

The New York Times reported on a 2006 study which found that even though protection from breast cancer varied among the types of tumor, exercise offered the most marked protection from the more aggressive tumors. A second study, also done in 2006, supported this finding.[131]

Several studies also suggested that more intense exercise is more protective against breast cancer. Exercising consistently throughout life gives the best protection. Exercise not only lowers a woman's chance of getting breast cancer, it can help those who have received chemotherapy for the disease fight off fatigue.[132]

Low-intensity exercise has a protective effect against colon cancer, according to the Nurses' Health Study and the American Cancer Society's Cancer Prevention Study II. Furthermore, a 2006 study found that people with colon cancer who exercise reduce their risk of a recurrence.[133]

Radiation and Sun

Ultraviolet radiation tanning beds and UV radiation were moved up to the highest cancer risk category by a World Health Organization agency. The comprehensive meta-analysis concluded that the risk of skin melanoma is increased by 75% when use of tanning devices starts before 30 years of age.[134]

Many of the more than 1 million skin cancers that are diagnosed every year could have been prevented by protecting the skin from the sun's rays and avoiding indoor tanning. The chances of getting skin cancer can be lowered by staying in the shade as much as you can, wearing a hat and shirt when you are in the sun, and using sunscreen.[135]

Smoking

Tobacco use accounts for 30% of all cancer deaths in the U.S., and for 87% of lung cancer death in particular. Not only does it affect the lungs, it can cause cancers of the mouth, lips, nose, sinuses, larynx, throat, esophagus, stomach, pancreas, kidney, bladder, uterine, and cervix, in addition to acute myeloid leukemia.[136]

Women who smoke two or more packs of cigarettes daily are 75% more likely to die from breast cancer, according to research by Eugenia E. Calle, Ph.D., of the American Cancer Society, Atlanta.[137]

Secondhand smoke causes 3,400 adults to die of lung cancer each year and also causes about 46,000 deaths from heart disease in people who are not current smokers.[138]

Cigarettes, cigars, pipes, and smokeless tobacco can all cause cancer and should not be used. People who already smoke should try to quit, as former smokers have less risk of cancer than do people who continue to smoke.[139] Cigar smoking causes cancers of the lung, mouth, larynx, esophagus, and possibly the pancreas.[140]

One study found that flavonoid intake, a reflection of fruit and vegetable consumption, was 21% lower in smokers than in nonsmokers. This may explain why smokers have a much higher incidence of lung cancer than nonsmokers.[141]

Stress

A study reported in the *British Medical Journal* found that severe psychological stress can increase the risk of breast cancer by 50%. Stress alters hormone production that, according to researchers, may lead to gene behavior that promotes the development of cancer.[142]

We know from experimental studies that stress is much more than psychological; it can have profound physical effects which can be quite harmful. For example, animals which are put under chronic, unrelieved stress have been found to have severe depression of their immune system, especially in terms of cellular immune response. This immune suppression can persist for a very long time. In addition, chronic stress can dramatically increase the formation of free radicals.[143]

Surgery and Anesthesia

It is well known that surgery and especially anesthesia are powerful suppressors of immune function. This level of immune suppression can give cancer a chance to invade and spread.[144]

Studies conducted in animals and humans suggest that the type of anesthesia used during surgery and the operation itself sap the immune system. According to Daniel Sessler, MD, senior author of a recent study, "Cancer surgery as done normally is bad for the immune system because the surgery itself, the anesthesia, and the opioids used to control pain all impair natural killer cell function."[145]

Trans Fats

Trans fats are present in meat and dairy products as well as in vegetable oils that have been chemically changed to improve their shelf life. Margarines and shortenings are the predominant sources of these fats. They are used in a variety of products such as cookies, crackers, potato and tortilla chips, cakes, non-dairy creamers, pizzas, donuts, and french fries.[146]

These fats raise total cholesterol. They may also be more cancer-promoting than other fats because of the disruption of the natural cell membranes in our bodies. An increase in the risk of colon cancer has been specifically linked with increased consumption of trans fats.[147]

Chapter 5:
The Diet-Cancer
Connection

*So many of us want a scapegoat… we do
not want to hear that our favorite foods
are a problem simply because of their
nutritional content.*

~ Mark Bittman

Up to now, we have discussed cancer as an epidemic. We have learned about carcinogens, the different types of cancer, and their risk factors. We have learned how cells mutate. But, you may be asking, how can we stop or slow down this epidemic? How can we decrease the number of people who get a cancer diagnosis each year? How can we protect ourselves and our families from this onslaught of disease?

Once you understand the growth of a tumor, you realize that early detection is probably a fallacy. If early detection is indeed a fallacy, we should be putting our efforts into prevention; and I think there is very good evidence that prevention can be accomplished through nutrition.

In this chapter, we are going to learn about some of the research behind the diet-cancer connection. Therefore, I hope you will begin to see that we can make a big impact against cancer not only for ourselves, but for our families and friends as well. If we use a low estimate that 35% of cancers could be prevented through diet, based on the figures in Chapter 1 we could be preventing nearly 200,000 deaths a year and over 500,000 new diagnoses. I think that would be a major victory in our "War on Cancer" and well worth pursuing!

I want to start off with a couple of stories before telling you about some laboratory studies. Then I want to tell you about the largest epidemiological study ever undertaken that will add substantial credibility to those lab experiments.

Dr. Neal Barnard tells the story of Anthony J. Sattilaro, MD, who wrote the book *Recalled by Life*. Tony was president of Methodist Hospital in Philadelphia. One day he had a routine chest x-ray and the radiologist found a puzzling density in the left side of his chest. More tests were ordered, and in the course of a few hours, Dr. Sattilaro went from being a busy doctor preoccupied with his work to being a patient with advanced cancer.[1]

Tony was only 46 and was told to get his affairs in order. He had an advanced form of prostate cancer which had metastasized to his lungs. Not long afterward, the pain took hold. As it worsened, he began to need narcotic painkillers to get through the day. Between the side effects of his medications and the cancer pain, he struggled to continue his work at the hospital.[2]

Dr. Barnard goes on to tell the story that Tony recounts in his book. After the burial of his father, who died of lung cancer, Dr. Sattilaro was driving back to Philadelphia on the New Jersey Turnpike. Deeply depressed, he uncharacteristically picked up two young hitchhikers who had just gotten out of macrobiotic cooking school. Tony tells the young men that he is living on borrowed time, and to his surprise he is told that his illness is curable if he will go on a strange vegetarian diet. A few days after their drive together, the young cooks mailed Dr. Sattilaro some information about macrobiotics and a macrobiotic teaching center in Philadelphia.[3]

Though highly skeptical, but with a sense of desperation and feeling as though he had nothing to lose, Dr. Sattilaro began eating meals at the macrobiotic center.[4]

A modern macrobiotic diet draws heavily on traditional Asian foods with generous amounts of rice and vegetables. Dairy products, meats, and sugary and refined foods are avoided.[5]

Tony followed the diet—with no Western indulgences whatsoever—and within three weeks his pain was gone and his energy returned and he was able to go back to work. A year later, the cancer was not showing up on any of the scans.[6]

Dr. Sattilaro stayed on the diet for a number of years, but eventually went off. Soon thereafter, his cancer returned and the pain enveloped him again. After he died, the question remained. Did his diet change make his cancer disappear? Had abandoning the diet caused it to return?[7]

Nathan Pritikin, diagnosed with leukemia in the early 1950s, was treated with chemotherapy, and had a remission of his symptoms. In 1958, at the age of 41, he was diagnosed with substantial coronary heart disease after a stress electrocardiogram. His cholesterol level was 300![8]

His cardiologists gave him the standard prescription of the day: stop all exercise, stop climbing stairs, take it easy, and take naps in the afternoon; but he knew he had to do something more if he wanted to live.[9]

After doing extensive research of population studies in the scientific literature, he figured he might have a chance of surviving if he could get his cholesterol reading down below 160. Pritikin became a vegetarian and started running three to four miles daily. Within two years his cholesterol had fallen to 120, and a new electrocardiogram showed that his coronary insufficiency had disappeared.[10]

After achieving such success in his own life, he was ready to help others. Over the next 25 years, he launched over 100 research projects and wrote 10 books on *The*

Pritikin Program, of which over three million books are still in print today.[11]

Pritikin died at the age of 70 of complications of his leukemia. His autopsy, as reported in the *New England Journal of Medicine*, showed that his arteries were free of any signs of heart disease. He is also on record as one of those who had lived the longest with that type of cancer.[12] After he died, the question remained: Did his diet change make his cancer disappear?

Let's continue with our hypothesis that there is a connection between diet and cancer by reviewing the literature.

In 1968, a research paper was published in India by Madhavan and Gopalan, describing an experiment involving two groups of laboratory rats. The first group of rats was given aflatoxin and then fed a diet containing 20% protein. The second group was given the same amount of aflatoxin and then fed a diet containing only 5% protein.[13]

Every single rat was predisposed to get liver cancer after being given aflatoxin. The result of this study was that all the rats fed the 20% protein diet did get liver cancer or precursor lesions but, amazingly, not a single rat fed the 5% protein diet got liver cancer or precursor lesions.[14]

Through more research, it has been found that lower protein intake can dramatically decrease tumor initiation at stage one; i.e., if you have been exposed to a carcinogen, you can actually decrease the number of mutations that might occur by eating less protein. And during the 10- to 20-year "promotion" stage, tumor growth can be turned on and off by dietary protein.[15] This is profoundly important—cancer growth can actually be reversed.[16]

In a 1978 journal article, Dr. Gio B. Gori stated that diet and nutrition appear to be related to the largest number of human cancers, second only to smoking.[17]

Sir Richard Doll and Sir Richard Peto, in a 1981 treatise, estimated that approximately 35% of all cancer mortality in the United States is related to diet. That 35% equals nearly 200,000 Americans who could be saved each year through changing their diet.[18]

In a 1987 study by Dunaif and Campbell, 10 groups of rats were administered increasing doses of aflatoxin, and then fed either 20% protein levels or 5% protein levels during the promotion period. In the animals fed the 20% level of protein, foci (precursor clusters of cells in the development of carcinomas) increased in number and size. However, in the animals fed 5% protein, there was no foci response, even when animals were given the maximum tolerated dose of aflatoxin.[19] The results were later repeated by Campbell and Youngman in 1991.[20]

The findings of these experiments are illustrated in the chart below.

Subjects	Carcinogen	Diet	Result
Rats – Group 1	Given high dose of aflatoxin	Fed 5% protein diet (casein)	Developed substantially less foci
Rats – Group 2	Given low dose of aflatoxin	Fed 20% protein diet (casein)	Developed substantially more foci

In other experiments, Youngman and Campbell dosed all animals with the same amount of carcinogen, then alternately fed either 5% or 20% dietary protein during the 12–week promotion stage. When animals were fed the 20% protein diet during periods 1 and 2, foci continued to enlarge. But when animals were switched to the low-protein diet at the beginning of period 3, there was a sharp decrease in foci development. And, when animals were subsequently switched back to the 20% protein diet during period 4, foci development was turned on once again.[21]

These experiments showed that, when subjects were given more or less protein at different stages of the progression, tumor growth could be turned "on" and "off" by varying the levels of protein in the animals' food. Those results were quite profound, and certainly convinced me that there is definitely a connection between diet and cancer.

As shown in the following table, foci growth could be changed, up and down, by switching the amount of protein being consumed.

Subjects	Carcinogen	First six weeks	Result	Next three weeks	Result	Last three weeks	Result
Group of Rats	All dosed with the same amount of aflatoxin	All fed 20% protein diet (casein)	Foci continued to enlarge	All switched to 5% protein diet (casein)	Sharp decrease in foci growth	All switched back to 20% protein diet (casein)	Foci growth was turned back on again

Other studies showed that an early carcinogenic exposure could be genetically remembered, but could lie dormant for many years while on a 5% protein diet, but could be "reawakened" by bad nutrition later.[22]

Experiments done in laboratories with rats can give rather dramatic results, but they are not humans. Unfortunately we cannot really do human experiments, but the next best thing would be population studies to see if the laboratory experiments can be duplicated.

During the 1980s and 1990s, a massive epidemiological study was conducted which compared the diets, lifestyle and disease characteristics of populations of 65 rural counties in China. Much of the initial funding came from the U.S. National Cancer Institute and the National Institutes of Health.[23] Other funding came from Oxford University, Cornell University, and the government of China. Professor T. Colin Campbell of Cornell led the first two major studies.

In 1981, the Chinese Academy of Medical Sciences published an *Atlas of Cancer Mortality* on the 1973–75 mortality rates for 14 different cancers in the 2392 counties of China. These maps showed that cancer was highly localized in specific geographic regions.[24]

Residents of these regions tended to live in the same areas all their lives and to consume the same diets unique to each area each and every year. Their diets (low in fat and high in dietary fiber and plant material) were in stark contrast to the rich diets of the Western countries.[25]

Within each of the 65 counties selected for the study, two villages were selected, and 50 families in each were randomly chosen for study. One adult from each of the 6,500 households (half men and half women) participated. Blood, urine, and food samples were obtained for later analysis, while questionnaires were filled out and 3-day diet information was recorded.[26]

A total of 367 items of information on these 6500 families eventually were judged to be reliable. The 1983–84 diet and lifestyle data included the 1973–75 mortality rates for about four dozen different kinds of cancers and other diseases.[27]

John Robbins, author of the book *Healthy at 100*, best describes the background of this immense project.

> The survey found that cancers were vastly more common in some parts of China than in others. This was of compelling interest for two reasons: first, because the difference in cancer rates between some Chinese counties was actually far greater than the difference between many of the world's nations; and second, because these differences were occurring in a country where 87 percent of the population belong to the same ethnic group (the Han people) and are genetically quite similar.[28]
>
> The difference in cancer rates between counties was staggering. Some counties, for example, had death rates from colon cancer that were twenty times greater than those of other counties. Similar differences were found for breast cancer, lung cancer, liver cancer, and many other forms of cancer.[29]
>
> The world medical community wanted to know what was going on in China. What would explain the fact that men in one part of China die from cancer of the esophagus 435 times more frequently than men in another part? And why was overall cancer

so much less common in China than in the United States and other Western nations?[30]

The China Project represented a once-in-the-history-of-humanity opportunity. In the 1980s, China was a perfect "living laboratory" for studying diet and disease patterns, unparalleled anywhere else in the world. This was because the Chinese still tended to spend their entire lives in the same area. Furthermore, these people had eaten food from the same area their whole lives.[31]

According to Dr. Campbell, "When we were done we had more than 8,000 statistically significant associations between lifestyle, diet and disease variables. We had a study that was unmatched in terms of comprehensiveness, quality and uniqueness. We had what the *New York Times* termed 'the Grand Prix of epidemiology.'"[32]

Chapter 6:
Steps to Prevent Cancer

Restlessness and discontent are the first necessities of progress.

~ Thomas A. Edison

Why isn't the diet connection to cancer more wide-spread? Is it because we would all rather have a miraculous "cure," like a pill or some magic procedure, or maybe a vaccine to just wipe it out?

Why won't your physician tell you to eat a plant-based diet?

In a recent lecture, Dr. John McDougall noted that many physicians will not talk to their female patients about drastically changing their diet because they assume they will not do it.[1]

"Yet," McDougall responds, "a woman will go through yearly mammograms, monthly breast self-exams, will allow a male physician to examine her breasts every year…she'll allow a biopsy, a lymph node removal, radiation, ovary removal, anti-estrogen drugs and chemotherapy…but she won't eat oatmeal?"[2]

If breast cancer treatments don't really work compared to survival, what's the harm in trying diet and lifestyle changes? Changing your diet will not make your hair fall out or make you vomit for a year. Adding exercise to your routine won't deform you. In fact, these diet and lifestyle changes will actually make you look better.[3]

Researchers at a recent breast cancer conference in Barcelona reported that up to a third of breast cancer cases in Western countries could be avoided if women ate less and exercised more.[4]

Michael Thun, MD, MS, vice president of epidemiology and surveillance research at the American Cancer Society, said, "What's interesting is that even without the potential benefits of early detection and treatment, at least one-third of cancer deaths are preventable."[5]

The World Health Organization predicts there will be a sharp increase in new cases of cancer diagnosed globally this year, making "a strong justification from a global perspective to focus on two main cancer-causing factors— tobacco and diet."[6]

Numerous epidemiological studies have shown that people who eat a lot of fruits and vegetables have much lower cancer rates than those who eat few or none. Scientists have used sophisticated instruments to look deep into the interior of cells, and have learned that various components of plants can affect cancer cells in such a way as to cause them to stop growing or even die.[7]

According to Dr. Campbell in *The China Study*, "There is a mountain of scientific evidence to show that the healthiest diet you can possibly consume is a high-carbohydrate diet."[8] We know that 99% of carbohydrates come from fruits, vegetables, and whole grains.[9] That means eat an apple, a zucchini or a plate of brown rice topped with beans and other vegetables.[10]

Based on all of my research, I think there are basically three steps to prevent, or reverse, the vast majority of cancers. I list those steps in the "short" version that follows. There is also a "long" version; not to replace the "short" version, but to add more detail to it—if you want to read it.

The Short Version

> **Diet**: Eat a whole-foods, plant-based diet (fresh vegetables and fruits, whole grain products like

brown rice and oatmeal, legumes, and nuts) with little or no added fat, salt, sugar, or processed food.

> **Exercise**: 15 to 45 minutes of moderate exercise every day.

> **Sunshine**: 15 minutes of sunshine every couple of days.

The Long Version

If you pay attention to the news media, you can hear a new prevention strategy each day; so for those of you who like things a bit more complicated, here's your list:

> **Eat sauerkraut.** A Finnish study found that the fermentation process involved in making sauerkraut produces several cancer-fighting compounds.[11]

> **Eat broccoli.** Steam it, eat it raw, or add it to soups and salads. A Spanish study found that microwaving broccoli destroys 97% of its flavonoids.[12]

> **Eat cruciferous vegetables.** Broccoli, cabbage, brussels sprouts, and cauliflower contain compounds called indoles which have been shown to break down estrogen into noncarcinogenic forms of the hormone.[13]

> **Eat dark, leafy greens.** This includes collard greens, kale, and spinach.[14]

> **Eat two Brazil nuts a day.** They are a rich source of selenium. A Harvard study of more than 1,000 men with prostate cancer found that those with the highest

blood levels of selenium were 48% less likely to develop advanced disease over 13 years than men with the lowest levels.[15]

> **Add garlic to everything you eat.** Garlic contains sulfur compounds that may stimulate the immune system's natural defenses against cancer, and may have the potential to reduce tumor growth.[16]

> **Eat tomatoes.** In animal studies, Japanese researchers described how lycopene suppressed the growth of breast cancers.[17]

> **Make pasta sauce with low-sodium, diced tomatoes.** The lycopene in the tomatoes protects against colon, prostate, and bladder cancers.[18]

> **Eat cooked tomatoes.** A Harvard Medical School study showed that men who ate cooked tomatoes several times weekly were less likely to have prostate cancer.[19]

> **Eat cantaloupe.** It's a great source of carotenoids, which are plant chemicals that have been shown to significantly reduce the risk of lung cancer.[20]

> **Mix some blueberries in your cereal each morning.** The antioxidants in blueberries help neutralize free radicals.[21]

> **Eat artichokes.** The silymarin in artichokes may help prevent skin cancer.[22]

> **Eat kiwifruit.** It contains cancer-fighting antioxidants; including vitamin C, vitamin E, lutein, and copper.[23]

> **Eat grapes.** They're great sources of resveratrol. Resveratrol is an antioxidant, anti-inflammatory substance found in the skin, seeds, and stems of the grape plant.[24]

> **Eat onions.** A diet high in onions may reduce the risk of prostate cancer by 50%. The effects are strongest when they're eaten raw or lightly cooked.[25]

> **Eat citrus fruits.** Australian researchers found that a daily dose of citrus may cut the risk of mouth, throat, and stomach cancers by half.[26]

> **Eat a diet high in vitamin C.** These foods include asparagus, berries, broccoli, cabbage, melons, cauliflower, citrus fruits, kale, kiwifruit, potatoes, spinach, and tomatoes.

> **Eat carrots.** The long-term consumption of diets rich in beta-carotene can reduce the risk of postmenopausal breast cancer.[27]

> **Eat superstar fruits.** These include citrus, berries and cherries.[28]

> **Choose cucumbers instead of pickles.** Studies find that pickled and smoked foods contain various carcinogens.[29]

> **Eat vegetables with high ORAC scores.** Kale, spinach, Brussels sprouts, alfalfa sprouts, broccoli flowers, beets, red bell peppers, onions, corn, and eggplant are top performers for their antioxidant power and oxygen radical absorbance capacity.[30]

> **Eat fruits with high ORAC scores.** Prunes, raisins, blueberries, blackberries, strawberries, raspberries, plums, oranges, red grapes and cherries are top performers for their antioxidant power and oxygen radical absorbance capacity.[31]

> **Don't eat french fries, potato chips, or baked sweets.** A potential cancer-causing compound called acrylamide forms when foods are baked, fried, or roasted.[32]

> **Avoid meat.** Meat enhances the production of insulin-like growth factor (IGF-1), and this enhances cancer cell growth.

> **Avoid dairy products.** Dairy products also enhance the production of IGF-1, which enhances cancer cell growth.[33] At least one study has shown that natural sugars in dairy products may raise the risk for ovarian cancer in some women.[34]

> **Consume whole food soy products like tofu, tempeh, soy milk, and edamame.** According to scientists from the Northern California Cancer Center, "Eating tofu regularly can almost halve a woman's chances of developing ovarian cancer."[35]

> **Don't eat processed soy products.** The synthetically manufactured foods can be just as harmful as animal products. Names for processed products include hydrolyzed soy protein, isolated soy protein, soy concentrates, textured vegetable protein, soy lecithin, soybean oil, etc.[36]

> **Eat more fiber.** Studies based on the work of Denis Burkitt found that adding a cup of red raspberries or a cup of beans to your diet each day could lower your long-term risk of colon cancer by 33%.[37]

> **Eat complex carbohydrates.** Unprocessed fresh fruits and vegetables and whole grain products like brown rice and oatmeal are exceptionally health-promoting.[38]

> **Eat whole grains.** Many epidemiologic studies suggest

that whole-grain consumption reduces the risk of developing cancers of the stomach, colon, mouth, gall-bladder, and ovaries.[39]

> **Avoid refined carbohydrates.** Refined carbohydrates are white flour, sugar, sugary cereals, white bread, candies, and sugar-laden soft drinks; they have absolutely no food value.[40]

> **Maintain a healthy body weight.** Keep your body mass index (BMI) score under 25. An elevated BMI has been shown to increase the risk of postmenopausal breast cancer.[41]

> **Cut down on fat.** This is an important first step in preventing cancer and in surviving it.[42] Many studies have shown that slimmer people are less likely to develop cancer, and trimming excess weight may also improve survival after cancer has been diagnosed.[43]

> **Reduce your consumption of omega-6 fats.** These include sunflower, safflower, corn, cottonseed , peanut, and soybean oils.[44]

> **Eliminate trans fats.** Partially hydrogenated oils are commonly found in vegetable shortening, some margarines, crackers, candies, baked goods, snack foods, fried foods, salad dressings, and many processed foods. If the ingredient list includes the words "shortening," "partially hydrogenated vegetable oil," or "hydrogenated vegetable oil," the food contains trans fat. Top nutritionists at Harvard have concluded that trans fat could be responsible for as many as 30,000 premature deaths per year.[45]

> **Keep your salt intake to a minimum.** Avoid highly processed and packaged foods, which contain excess salt. A salty diet is linked to stomach cancer.[46]

> **Eat mushrooms and drink green tea.** Chinese women who ate mushrooms and drank green tea significantly cut their risk of breast cancer, and the severity of the cancer in those who did develop it.[47]

> **Eat red grapes and dark chocolate.** They have ingredients that starve cancer while feeding bodies, according to Angiogenesis Foundation head William Li.[48]

> **Drink papaya leaf tea.** Researchers have said that papaya leaf extract and its tea have dramatic cancer-fighting properties against a broad range of tumors, including those of the cervix, breast, liver, lung, and pancreas.[49]

> **Drink water.** A major study published in the *New England Journal of Medicine* in 1996 found that men who drank six 8-ounce glasses of water every day slashed their risk of bladder cancer in half. Another study found that women who drank water reduced their risk of colon cancer.[50]

> **Drink tea.** A chemical in green tea called EGCG is a powerful antioxidant.[51]

> **Have a beer.** Don't overdo it, as drinking more than one or two alcoholic drinks a day can increase your risk of some cancers. However, beer seems to protect against the *H. pylori* bacteria, which is known to cause ulcers and is possibly linked to stomach cancer.[52]

> **Minimize your intake of alcohol.** Your risk of developing mouth, throat, esophagus, kidney, liver, and breast cancers increases with the amount of alcohol you drink and the length of time you've been drinking regularly. Even a moderate amount of drinking—two drinks a day if you're a man or one drink a day if you're a woman, and one drink a day regardless of your sex if you're over 65—may increase your risk.[53]

> **Get a little sunshine.** All you need is about 15 minutes every couple of days to increase your levels of vitamin D.[54]

> **Use sunscreen.** Use at least 1.5 ounces and rub it all over your body to protect yourself from the cancer-causing UV rays of the sun. Repeat every two hours.[55]

> **Don't use sunscreen.** Some scientists studying cancer have come to virtually the opposite conclusion; that is, the use of sunscreen chemicals may be increasing the incidence of cancer due to their free-radical-generating properties, and because the chemicals most commonly used in sunscreens have strong estrogenic actions.[56]

> **Take a walk.** According to a study from the Fred Hutchinson Cancer Research Center in Seattle, all you need is a 30–minute walk to reduce your levels of estrogen, a hormone that contributes to breast cancer. Another study linked four hours a week of walking or hiking with cutting the risk of pancreatic cancer in half. The benefits are probably related to improved insulin metabolism.[57]

> **Learn to live with weeds.** By using commercial pesticides on your lawn, you may increase your risk of cancer.[58]

> **Buy clothes that don't have to be dry cleaned.** Many dry cleaners still use a chemical called perchloroethylene, which has been found to cause kidney and liver damage. If you dry-clean your clothes, take them out of the plastic bag and let them air for an hour before wearing them.[59]

> **Avoid tanning beds.** Go for a spray-on tan, as there is no evidence that this type of product increases your risk of skin cancer.[60]

> **Use tanning beds.** In an opposing view, indoor tanning machines emit the same spectrum UVB radiation as sunlight. People living in areas where sunlight is limited can use an indoor tanning bed at least once a week to raise their vitamin D levels.[61]

> **Keep up with your friends.** A study from the State University of New York at Stony Brook found that men with high levels of stress and those with less satisfying contacts with friends and family members had higher levels of PSA in their blood, a marker for the development of prostate cancer.[62]

> **Maintain a positive mental attitude.** Engage in self-nurturing behaviors regularly. Develop rich, warm relationships with friends and family. Get adequate sleep.[63]

> **Minimize exposure to pharmacologic estrogens.** Your lifetime exposure to estrogen plays a fundamental role in the development of breast cancer.[64]

> **Don't use tobacco.** All types of tobacco put you on a collision course with cancer.[65]

> **Get immunized.** Certain cancers are associated with viral infections that can be prevented with immunizations. Talk to your doctor about immunization against hepatitis B or HPV.[66]

> **Use a condom and stick to one partner.** The more sexual partners a woman has, the greater her risk of contracting HPV, which causes cervical cancer. An unfaithful husband also increases her risk.[67]

> **Avoid risky behaviors.** Viruses can be transmitted sexually or by using contaminated needles.[68]

> **Get screened.** Death is prevented by finding changes before they are cancer. Tests that can find those superficial changes include Pap smears for cervical cancer; sigmoidoscopy or double-contrast barium enema for colon polyps; oral cancer screenings for leukoplakia; and body screenings by a dermatologist to check for melanoma.[69]

> **Avoid using cell phones.** Studies led by Professor Lennart Hardell in Sweden found significantly increased risk of brain tumors from 10 or more years of cell phone or cordless phone use.[70] Steps to reduce exposure to cell phone radiation include:

>> Avoid holding a cell phone close to the head for extended periods.

>> Use a wired headset or send messages by texting.

> Keep the cell phone away from your body, including pockets.

> Avoid using a cell phone in a moving vehicle or a building as that tends to increase the power and the radiation required.

> Use the cell phone like an answering machine by keeping it off until the user is ready to return calls.

> Use a corded, landline phone whenever possible.

> Children under 18 should not be allowed to use a cell phone except in an emergency.

> Never sleep with a cell phone under your pillow.[71]

> **Avoid flights with Wi-Fi.** Wi-Fi in the sky adds a significant additional source of non-ionizing radiation to the flying environment.[72]

Chapter 7:
You Can Change Your Lifestyle

*There is enough evidence now
that doctors should be discussing
the option of pursuing
dietary change as a potential path to
cancer treatment and prevention.*

~ T. Colin Campbell, PhD,
The China Study

If you decide that you believe the evidence I've put before you, and if you decide that you want to know more, and if you plan to follow up with the background of evidence I've brought to you, you may decide to change.

And this will be the biggest stumbling block. You may know in the back of your head that changing your lifestyle is exactly what you need to do, but it would be so much easier if cancer were like food poisoning. You eat a spoiled food and within 24 hours you become violently ill. If that has ever happened to you, you have probably not eaten that food or gone to that place again. It's so much easier to change your behavior if the cause and effect are immediate.

Even gaining weight is a very slow process. What if you ate that box of doughnuts one day and the next day you were 30 pounds heavier? That would probably get your attention a lot more than the one pound a month you normally put on. At that rate it takes you two and a half years to gain that same 30 pounds and you just get used to it. You start thinking that's your "normal" weight, which is the mass your bones were meant to hold.

At least if you want to see how much weight you've gained, you can find an old photo of you at a normal weight and compare with one taken now. If you think you've been fat all your life, go back as far as you need to find that photo of you *before* you were fat—even if you have to go back to age three. Some of you will only have to go back to high school or college, or when you were in the military or first married.

Another reason it's so hard to change is that we have always used food as a reward. Mothers begin taking their babies to get ice cream for a little treat or planning birthday parties or sleepovers for their kids and plying them with soft drinks, pizzas, doughnuts, cookies, and birthday cakes. If children eat their meals, they are rewarded with a sweet, caloric dessert. Even as adults, we reward ourselves with Starbucks or a trip to the new cupcake store.

Emotionally, we are programmed to reward ourselves with junk food. Did you know that cheese consumption for Americans has gone up from 3 pounds a year to over 10 pounds a year? Cheese is 70% fat—mostly saturated fat.[1] What do you think that does to a child?

Sugar, caffeine, alcohol, salt, and fat are all extremely addictive. Once we get used to eating or drinking those things, our brains don't want us to let them go. We can have pains of withdrawal and lack of serotonin. Those cravings are real and sometimes can be as powerful as those of an alcoholic or drug addict.

One reason for the popularity of the Atkins diet is because it's easy and it encourages us to eat the foods we have come to love. Dr. McDougall laughingly says, "The Atkins diet is easy. Drive through a fast food restaurant, order a burger, throw away the bun, eat the burger and you're on the Atkins diet."[2]

Every successful lifestyle change you make must become a habit. If, every time you are presented with both healthy and unhealthy choices, you think, "I know I shouldn't, but maybe I can do it just once," you know it has not become a habit.

Habits just make choices easier. If you have made a habit of brushing your teeth each night before you go to bed, you just do it. You don't stand at the sink each night and say, "I know I should brush my teeth, but maybe I won't tonight."

If you have a habit of jumping out of bed each morning and going for a walk or going to the gym, you just do it. You don't agonize each morning as to whether you will or won't today. If you have a habit of stopping at Starbucks each morning for a 330–calorie Caffè Mocha with nonfat milk, you just do it.

How do you exchange a "bad" habit for a "good" one? First and foremost, you have to decide that it's worth it to you. If you think you might "try" to be a vegan, you will only be a vegan for a few days because you will wear yourself out with the decisions you are having to make each time you get ready to eat or drink something.

If you decide to become a vegan or a vegetarian, you will take a lot of guff for it from many of your friends and relatives. That's why it has to come from the power of your conviction first and foremost. If you feel that it's the right thing, the hard part won't be deciding on a daily basis. The hard part will be learning new ways of cooking and eating. But once you are convinced, you will find ways to make it work.

Think about the first time you realized that exercise was going to be part of your life. That happened for me in 1972 when Kenneth Cooper wrote the book *Aerobics* and then his wife Millie wrote *Aerobics for Women*. I realized that it was something I wanted to do, so I decided to do it. I then had to figure out if I would run in the dark before taking the kids to school or if I would sign up for a Jazzercise class a couple of times a week or whether I would join a tennis league. Those details just had to be worked out and made into habits, because my decision to exercise had already been made.

Many of you have heard the old joke: Eating a healthy diet may not actually make you live longer, but it sure feels that way. In the beginning, you may repeat that joke yourself, but as you continue to change your habits, you will enjoy the benefits so much that you won't want to go back to your old lifestyle.

Not only will this way of life improve your odds of keeping many cancers at bay, but it will also improve your odds of keeping obesity, heart disease, type 2 diabetes, osteoporosis, multiple sclerosis, and other autoimmune diseases at bay as well. An exciting side effect of this lifestyle will be watching as your body gets back to its ideal size.

When cancer researchers started to look for links between diet and cancer, one of the most noticeable findings was that people who avoided meat were less likely to develop the disease. Large studies in Germany and Japan showed that vegetarians were about 40 percent less likely to develop cancer compared to meat eaters.[3]

One of the secrets to this healthy lifestyle is swapping out empty-calorie meals loaded with unhealthy fats for nutrient-dense, antioxidant-rich alternatives.[4]

What Can I Eat?

You can eat vegetables, fruits, whole grains, and

starch-based foods. Starch-based foods include the following:

- ⟩ Potatoes
- ⟩ Sweet potatoes
- ⟩ Frozen hash browns
- ⟩ Brown rice
- ⟩ Wild rice
- ⟩ Bulgur wheat
- ⟩ Couscous
- ⟩ Oats
- ⟩ Quinoa
- ⟩ Rye
- ⟩ Corn
- ⟩ Garbanzo beans
- ⟩ Lima beans
- ⟩ Black beans
- ⟩ Great Northern beans
- ⟩ Red kidney beans
- ⟩ Navy beans
- ⟩ Pinto beans
- ⟩ Cannellini beans
- ⟩ Black-eyed peas
- ⟩ Split green peas

- ❧ Pastas (egg-free)

- ❧ Rice noodles

- ❧ Squashes

- ❧ Stone ground bread (oil-free, dairy-free, egg-free)

- ❧ Whole wheat pita bread

- ❧ Whole grain cereals (with shortest list of ingredients, oil-free, additive-free; good choices include Shredded Wheat, Grape-Nuts, Corn Flakes)

- ❧ Popcorn (with no added ingredients)

- ❧ Rice cakes (with no added fats or oils)

- ❧ Crackers (whole grain, with no added fats or oils)

- ❧ Pretzels (no added fats or oils)

What About Fats?

All fats, saturated and unsaturated, are involved in the growth of certain kinds of cancer cells. Scientific studies done on animals have shown that a higher consumption of fats will produce a higher incidence of cancer. The unsaturated fats in vegetable oils like corn oil, safflower oil, and margarines are the fats that most promote cancer. Vegetable oils, just like animal fats, are extremely fattening because of their high calorie content.[5]

People on vegan diets often replace meat and dairy products with soybeans and products derived from soybeans such as tofu, soy cheese, soy milk, miso, and tempeh. Soybeans are an excellent source of protein, but they contain far too much fat for regular use by most people. Tofu is a rich, high-fat, low-fiber food that should be used sparingly.[6]

High-fat plant foods like nuts, avocados, coconuts, and olives should be used as special treats. Vegetarians who are overweight and greasy-skinned are usually those whose diet is filled with these high-fat plant foods. Athletes, children, and pregnant women who may need to eat more calories may be able to eat these foods in moderation.[7]

Many people try to trim fat from their diets by switching from beef to chicken. But chicken has nearly as much fat as beef.[8]

Fat Content of Various Foods
(% of calories from fat)

- Leanest Beef   29%
- Skinless Chicken Breast   23%
- Sea Trout   32%
- White Tuna   16%
- Broccoli   8%
- Beans   4%
- Sweet Potato   1% [9]

What About Protein?

Protein excess is a real problem in developed societies. When the protein content of the diet exceeds 15% of its calories, the body's liver and kidneys are burdened with the task of removing the excessive amounts. Human breast milk is only 5% protein and it is the healthiest food for babies. Other protein amounts include: beef, with 25% protein; rice, with 8% protein; oranges, with 8%; potatoes, with 11%; and beans, with 26%.[10]

What About Vitamin Deficiencies?

The only possible deficiency in a vegan diet could be vitamin B_{12}. The average American has stored so much vitamin B_{12} in his body's tissues, and the vitamin is used so slowly that 20 to 30 years must pass before he will run out of it. To be safe and avoid this risk, after you've been off meats for three years, or if you're pregnant or a nursing mother, take 5 micrograms per day of a vitamin B_{12} supplement.[11]

What About Salt?

If you are eating a diet of healthy ingredients like starches and vegetables, you are eating a diet that is already low in sodium. If that is the case, adding a little salt to your foods will not cause you any trouble. However, 80% of the salt consumed by most Americans is intermingled with our processed foods. That's why scientific research incriminates salt; it is mixed up in any diet research with things like bacon grease, cheese, and hamburgers.[12]

The overpowering taste of salt actually tricks us into eating foods that normally repulse human beings because it disguises the awful tastes of animal flesh and cow's milk secretions. If you can give up your salt-laden foods such as breakfast burritos and those monster burgers, you can then add salt to your healthy starches and vegetables without worry.[13]

What About Fish and Chicken?

Red meat has been getting all the attention, but all animal foods contain exceedingly high levels of cholesterol. Being near the top of the food chain, they are all usually contaminated with pesticides, herbicides, drugs, and other toxic chemicals. Animal foods that contain high levels of cholesterol include beef, chicken, lamb, lobster, haddock, mackerel, pork, trout, turkey, veal, eggs, shrimp, crab, and liver.[14]

Much of the chicken feed used in our country even contains arsenic! The arsenic additive promotes the growth of blood vessels in chicken so that the meat appears pinker at the grocery store. That arsenic does the same thing to human cells, fueling a growth process known as angiogenesis, which can be a first step in human diseases such as cancer.[15]

Chicken also contains arachidonic acid, as explained by Dr. Andrew Weil. Arachidonic acid (AA) is a pro-inflammatory fatty acid that is found only in animal products.

Dr. Weil explains that, "heart disease and Alzheimer's—among many other diseases—begin as inflammatory processes. The same hormonal imbalance that increases inflammation also increases cell proliferation and the risk of malignant transformation."

We are discovering that inflammation is the key in so many of the diseases that plague us. So when you eat meat—and Dr. Weil points out that even chicken is full of arachidonic acid—you are stoking the fires of the disease process. It doesn't matter if the chicken is free-range or the beef is grass-fed. The offending fatty acid is natural and inherent in the meat.[16]

What About Food Additives?

In laboratory studies, there has been some observation that glutamate from food additives can enter the brain and increase the growth and aggressiveness of glioma-type brain tumors.[17] Glutamate is found in many processed foods, so read the labels. Regular and low-fat dairy products have high concentrations of glutamate.[18] It also occurs naturally in portobello mushrooms and is released when they are cooked.[19]

Carrageenan is a food additive in ice cream, yogurt, cottage cheese, and other processed food products, including some brands of soy milk. If you have been diagnosed with cancer, it might be wise to limit your intake of carrageenan.[20]

What About Red Wine?

Some researchers are looking at whether red wine may offer some protection against cancer because of resveratrol, which is an antioxidant. In animal studies, resveratrol has shown to slow down the growth of cancer cells. However, drinking too much alcohol increases the risk of some cancers, high blood pressure, high triglycerides, liver damage, obesity, mental illness, accidents, and many other health conditions. Of course, if you are pregnant or have liver disease, it is better to forego all alcoholic drinks.[21]

What About Fiber?

An average American gets only 10–15 grams of fiber per day. Health authorities would like to see that number rise significantly. A good goal to reach for is 40 grams per day.[22] Generally speaking, the most fiber-rich foods are beans and vegetables, followed by fruits and whole grains.[23]

Food	Grams of Fiber
Beans (1/2 cup)	7
Soy milk (1 cup)	3
Tofu (1/2 cup)	3
Vegetables (1/2 cup)	4
Lettuce (1/2 cup)	2
Potato (with skin)	4
Potato (without skin)	2
Fruit (one medium)	3
Fruit juice (1 cup)	1
Whole grain breads (1 slice)	1
Whole grain cooked pasta (1 cup)	2
Brown rice (1 cup)	3
White rice (1 cup)	1
Cooked oatmeal (1 cup)	4
Ready-to-eat cereals (1 cup)	3
Highly processed or colored cereals (1 cup)	1
Bran (1 cup)	8
Meat, poultry, or fish	0
Eggs or dairy products	0
Sodas, water	0

Animal products don't have any fiber. That is why people who center their diets on those foods often struggle
with constipation. On the other hand, plant products in
their natural state have quite a lot of fiber, which is why
vegetarians rarely have any need for laxatives.[24]

Among the most important themes to emerge from
research has been that foods influence the hormones that
fuel cancer growth. For example, diets high in fiber and
low in fat tend to reduce the amount of estrogens (female
sex hormones) circulating in the bloodstream. This taming
of estrogens seems to reduce the likelihood that cancer
cells will multiply or spread.[25]

What About Calcium?

Calcium is an essential nutrient. Good calcium sources
include beans, broccoli, collard greens, kale, sweet potatoes, soy milk, rice milk, almond milk, oat milk, and cal-
cium-fortified juices. Eating lots of fruits and vegetables,
limiting salt intake, and excluding animal proteins will help
your body retain calcium.[26]

What About Fatty Acids?

Fatty acids are simply components of fats. There are
two essential fatty acids that you need to get from your
diet because the body cannot manufacture them.[27]

> ⯈ Omega-3: Called alpha-linolenic acid (ALA). It
> is found in flax seed, walnuts, wheat germ, and
> dark green, leafy vegetables.

> ❧ Omega-6: Called linoleic acid (LA). You can get linoleic acid from sunflower seeds, safflower seeds, corn, pumpkin seeds, sesame seeds, tahini, and almost any kind of nuts.[28]

The body constructs hormones from these fatty acids. In general, the two acids have opposite effects. Those from omega-6 fatty acids tend to *increase* inflammation (an important component of the immune response), blood clotting, and cell proliferation. Those from omega-3 fatty acids *decrease* those functions. Both families of hormones must be in balance to maintain optimum health.[29]

Most Americans now get far too much of the omega-6s and not enough of the omega-3s. This dietary imbalance may explain the rise of such diseases as asthma, coronary heart disease, many forms of cancer, autoimmunity and neurodegenerative diseases; all of which are believed to stem from inflammation in the body.[30]

You can cut down on omega-6 levels by reducing consumption of processed and fast foods and polyunsaturated vegetable oils (corn, peanut, sunflower, safflower, soy, canola, and cottonseed, for example).[31]

Can Children Eat This Way?

When you are a mother, you are never really
alone in your thoughts.
A mother always has to think twice,
once for herself and once for her child.

~ Sophia Loren

Children raised on vegetables, fruits, whole grains, and legumes grow up slimmer and healthier, and they live longer than their meat-eating friends.[32]

Children can certainly enjoy this new lifestyle with you. A low-fat, plant-based diet which is based around unrefined starches, vegetables, and fruits is the healthiest diet for men, women, and children (after the age of 2 years). From birth to six months, babies should be exclusively breast-fed. After six months, solid foods in the form of starches, vegetables, and fruits are added in increasing amounts; and breast milk is continued until the child is at least 2 years of age.[33]

If you have any doubts about a healthy plant-based diet, you just have to look around. Children on diets with lots of ice cream, milk, hot dogs, egg muffins, and chicken nuggets are fat and sick. The obvious signs and symptoms are snotty noses, ear infections, stomach aches, and headaches. They are also probably constipated.[34]

You will be able to include your children in your new lifestyle, but you will have to speak to them in age-appropriate terms and you will have to model the behaviors for them.

Whenever my granddaughter stays with us, she adapts beautifully to our lifestyle. However, her mother tends to think (like most American mothers do) that you are "depriving" children if you take away their macaroni and cheese or their ice cream. It may be a subtle belief, but it comes through loud and clear to the child.

The foods we eat as children are those that we become addicted to.[35]

Very young children may need a slightly higher fat intake than adults do. In moderation, healthful fat sources include soybean products, avocados, and nut butters.[36] Children also need to take a vitamin B_{12} supplement of 5 micrograms per day.[37]

Growing children also need iron, which is found in a variety of beans and green, leafy vegetables. The vitamin C in vegetables and fruits enhances iron absorption when these foods are eaten along with an iron-rich food. One example is an iron-rich bean burrito eaten with vitamin C-rich tomato salsa.[38]

What if I Already Have Cancer?

It turns out that many foods which help prevent cancer in the first place also seem to help us beat the disease when it has struck.[39]

We tend to think of cancer as something that only surgery, radiation, or chemotherapy can control; and even they often fall short.[40]

If you have been diagnosed with cancer, realize that foods can influence the course of the disease once it has started.[41]

The body heals, but sometimes it can't keep up with the damage. Therefore, you must stop the damage. Stop the toxins. Stop the toxic foods of the rich American diet. And then the body will be able to do what it does naturally. It will heal.[42]

In 1980, researchers found that lung cancer patients who were smokers, and who kept smoking after their diagnosis, died much more often. Those who were over 65 and quit smoking lived twice as long.[43]

Even after you get sick, you ought to stop what made you sick. If you get breast cancer and you're overweight, you die twice as fast. If you have high cholesterol, you die faster. If you have high estrogen levels in the blood, you die faster.[44]

One way to assure adequate absorption of the cancer-suppressing nutrients found in produce for near-terminal cancer patients is to grind them up in a blender or to use a juicer.[45]

Fourteen of seventeen studies show a positive relationship between more plant foods and survival. Women with breast cancer who changed their diet lived longer.[46]

In many laboratory experiments, food was found to turn cancer growth "on" or "off." It has been estimated that as many as 60%–70% of all cancers are related to your diet. You don't want to continue eating the same foods that possibly led to your cancer in the first place.[47]

Experts say the focus must shift to changing behaviors like diet and physical activity. Those comments are added to a series of findings that lifestyle changes in other areas such as smoking and sun exposure can have a significant effect on all sorts of cancer rates.[48]

Michelle Holmes, a cancer expert at Harvard University, said people might wrongly think their chances of getting cancer are more dependent on their genes than their lifestyle.[49]

Many breast cancers are fueled by estrogen, a hormone produced in fat tissue. So experts suspect that the fatter a woman is, the more estrogen she's likely to produce. Even in slim women, exercise can help reduce the cancer risk by converting more of the body's fat into muscle.[50]

Foods influence the effects of estrogen. When a woman begins a low-fat, high-fiber diet, the amount of estrogen in her blood drops almost immediately. In a matter of weeks, the amount in her bloodstream drops by 15%–50%.[51]

The same phenomenon occurs in men. Men have estrogen in their blood, too—and as men cut the fat and increase fiber in their diets, the amounts of both estrogen and testosterone tend to fall.[52]

Any discussion of weight and breast cancer is considered sensitive because some people may misconstrue that the medical establishment is blaming victims for getting breast cancer. Victims themselves may also feel guilty, wondering just how much the issue of weight factored into their own cancer case.[53]

It is natural that concerns like these will cross our minds. The fact is, some people do their very best to live in a healthy manner and still develop cancer. And you may have known people who smoked, drank heavily, and ate with abandon and yet managed to live to a ripe old age.[54]

Don't focus on blame, but on what foods can do for you in the present.[55] In order to reduce cancer risk or effectively alter its course, dietary changes have to be significant.[56]

Should I Go with Conventional Treatments?

If you do get cancer, listen to your doctors, ask a lot of questions about recovery rates and survival rates for the various treatments, and then try to take some time to think about your options. If survival statistics for painful, disfiguring treatments aren't very good, you will have to make the decision as to whether those treatments are best for you.

Minimal treatments are sometimes best. If you have prostate cancer, you may want to do watchful waiting. Treatment options for prostate cancer basically give you the choice of being incontinent or impotent for the rest of your life. Much of the time, treatment has nothing to do with survival.[57]

Surgery, radiation, and/or chemotherapy do show substantial benefits for childhood cancers, testicular cancer, leukemia, and lymphoma.[58]

If you have breast cancer, you will want to get the lump out, but when it comes to tumors deep inside the body like breast or prostate cancer, there are very few other effective treatments.[59]

In a study reported at a recent breast cancer conference in Barcelona, it was found that, for some women, having a breast removed once they have been diagnosed with cancer doesn't always mean they'll live longer. More conservative treatment with chemotherapy and hormonal therapy is a very reasonable alternative. This should give recently diagnosed breast cancer patients a bit of breathing room.[60]

Standard cancer treatments often fail to eradicate cancer and can actually make it worse, according to Dr. Max Wicha, founder of the University of Michigan's Comprehensive Cancer Center. Even when chemotherapy and radiation cause tumors to shrink dramatically, the cancer stem cells that create those rapidly dividing tumor cells grow more slowly, and are therefore less susceptible to conventional therapies.[61]

It's Time to Change Your Diet

In order to reduce cancer risk or effectively alter its course, your dietary changes need to be significant. Studies have shown that modest changes in diet do little or nothing.[62]

As we have seen, there is a large body of evidence that foods definitely influence the hormones that drive cancer. This does not mean that patients should ignore other treatments, but it is important to also take advantage of the power that foods do have.[63]

In lab studies, when a very potent carcinogen is put into the body, the rate at which it causes problems can be controlled by nutrition. If you eat a Western-type diet, you will actually increase the rate that the chemical carcinogens form products in your body that cause cancer.[64]

Dr. Campbell reiterates that animal protein is the most carcinogenic substance we consume because 90%–95% of our exposure to environmental chemicals comes from eating animal products.[65]

Changing your diet can be a very difficult thing to do at any time, especially if you are suddenly classified as "sick." For a person used to living on barbecued ribs, french fries, and soft drinks, a change to eating fresh vegetables, fruits, and whole grains can be considered quite drastic.[66]

There are strong indications that if cancer patients begin to follow a strict diet regimen at the time of their original diagnosis and continue to follow it for life, most recurrences of cancer can be avoided.[67]

By improving your general nutrition, you will have a lot more energy, greater endurance, and far fewer complications associated with your treatments. Most patients feel a greater sense of well-being once they establish better eating habits. In addition, they begin to feel that they, not their cancer, are in control.[68]

Is There an Easy Way to Get Started?

To ensure that good foods will be available when you need them, you might try something like a Saturday or Sunday ritual. This is when you set aside a few hours to plan your weekly menu, make your list, go grocery shopping, and then put away the food. Because you are now purchasing more fresh foods, you will need to take the time to clean out your refrigerator before adding the new produce.

You can double-cook your dinner each night to insure that you have leftovers for a healthy lunch the next day. If you wish to be healthy and lean, you will need to remove all foods not conducive to those goals from your home. If you love to have a dish of ice cream before bed each evening, you will want to rid your freezer of ice cream so the temptation is removed.

Changing to a plant-based diet will cause changes in the pattern and consistency of your bowel movements. You will no longer be constipated. Gas is common and can be embarrassing as you add more vegetables, beans, and whole grains to your diet. You can take Beano®, a digestive enzyme that helps to reduce the gas caused by beans. It may take a few weeks for your digestive tract to get used to the change.

Chapter 8:
Questions You May Ask

*The great enemy of the truth
is very often not the lie—deliberate,
contrived and dishonest—but the
myth—persistent,
persuasive and unrealistic.*

~ John F. Kennedy

Once my friends and family heard that I was no longer eating animal protein, all of those well-known myths would spring to their minds and I was asked the same questions many times over.

- ❧ "Where do you get your protein?"

- ❧ "Where do you get your calcium?"

- ❧ "Do you eat organic foods?"

- ❧ "Do you eat fish or take fish oil?"

- ❧ "Do you take supplements?"

- ❧ "What if I have a family history of cancer?"

- ❧ "Are there any objective ways to determine if I'm on the right track?"

"Where do you get your protein?"

When discussing food sources of protein, nutritionists often speak in terms of "complete" and "incomplete" proteins. Foods that provide complete protein are those that include all of the essential amino acids, while foods that provide some or none of the essential amino acids are said to be incomplete.[1]

Eggs, dairy foods, meat, fish, and poultry are typically considered to be complete proteins. Vegetarians, and especially vegans, often do not have a source of complete protein in their diets, but they can easily obtain all of the essential amino acids by eating a variety of beans, grains, nuts, seeds, and vegetables.[2]

The idea that we must get our protein from meat is a well-known myth. Third world nations all over the globe who get enough calories in their diets eat little or no meat; yet many of them are in excellent health from eating only plant protein.[3]

It's easy to get all the protein we need without eating meat as we can get the amino acids we need from almost all foods.[4] Nearly every food has enough protein in it to supply us with the necessary amino acids—if we eat enough of it—to get a day's worth of calories, except for fruits, sugars, fats, and oils.[5]

The following vegan-friendly foods are loaded with protein: lentils, black beans, pinto beans, kidney beans, garbanzo beans, navy beans, almonds, pistachios, pumpkin seeds, almond butter, peanut butter, and hemp seeds. Just one serving of lentils mixed with one serving of hemp seeds gives you around 20 grams of complete protein. In addition, it is a nice balance of protein, carbohydrates, and healthy fat.[6]

According to the U.S. Recommended Dietary Allowance (RDA) for protein consumption, we should be getting about 10%–15% of our energy from protein. According to the World Health Organization (WHO), the U.S. RDA protein diet standards may be overestimated. The WHO puts our dietary protein needs more conservatively at about half of the U.S. government minimum levels.[7]

Because the average American's diet actually contains 15%–16% protein, most of us are getting too much. In laboratory experiments, scientists could turn cancer (tumor) growth off or on by changing the level of protein in the diet.[8]

In experimental studies of rats with liver cancer, most of the rats that were given diets of only 5% protein lived long lives; yet 100% of the rats that were given diets of 20% protein died at an early age. In those experiments, the protein source used was casein, a milk protein.[9]

Even athletes can grow big and strong on plant-based diets, according to strength and conditioning instructor Mike Mahler. According to Mahler, "Just because the pot-smoking hippie vegetarian in Venice Beach, CA, looks like he has not eaten in a month, does not mean that every vegan does. I have the strength and size to back up the fact that you can get strong and have a muscular body on a vegan diet and I am far from being the only one."[10]

"Where do you get your calcium?"

Why do nations like Denmark, Holland, Norway, and Sweden, with the highest rates of bone disease, also have the highest milk consumption rates?[11]

American women are told to consume 1,000 milligrams per day of calcium. The Inuit Eskimos consume 3,500 milligrams of calcium each day, and by age 40 are crippled.[12]

Mark Hegsted, retired Harvard professor of nutrition, believes we get too much calcium.[13]

In an article in the *Journal of Nutrition* he writes, "Hip fractures are more frequent in populations where dairy products are commonly consumed and calcium intakes are relatively high. Is there any possibility that this is a causal relationship?"[14]

There are more hip fractures in populations who eat dairy products and meats.[15]

Plenty of calcium is available in a wide range of plant foods, including beans and leafy vegetables. As long as you stay away from refined carbohydrates like sugary cereals, candies, plain pastas, and white breads, you should have no problem with calcium deficiency.[16]

It's not how much calcium you eat, but how much you prevent from leaving your bones, according to Dr. Breslau. In 1988, N.A. Breslau in the *Journal of Clinical Endocrinology* identified the relationship between protein-rich diets and calcium metabolism, noting that protein caused calcium loss.[17]

A 1994 study published in the *American Journal of Clinical Nutrition* found that animal proteins cause calcium to be leached from the bones and excreted in the urine.[18]

Dean Ornish, MD, writes, "The real cause of osteoporosis in this country is not insufficient calcium intake, it is excessive excretion of calcium in the urine. Even calcium supplementation is often not enough to make up for the increased calcium excretion. Vegetarians, in contrast, excrete much less calcium, and this is why they have very low rates of osteoporosis even though their dietary intake of calcium is lower than those on a meat-eating diet."[19]

Consuming dairy foods can increase the risk of prostate cancer.[20] From a 2001 Harvard review of the literature: "men with the highest dairy intakes had approximately double the risk of total prostate cancer."[21]

"Do you eat organic foods?"

The federal government began certifying foods as "organic" under Title 21 of the 1990 Farm Bill; and according to Mark Bittman, "Americans love the idea." Bittman writes in a *New York Times* article, "the truth is that most Americans eat so badly—we get 7 percent of our calories from soft drinks, more than we do from vegetables; the top food group by caloric intake is 'sweets'; and one-third of the nation's adults are now obese—that the organic question is a secondary one."[22]

Bittman continues, "There are cancer-causing chemicals such as acrylamide (found in processed or fried foods like potato chips) which have been linked to cancer in experimental studies. But we assume that if we could effectively remove this chemical from potato chips, they would be safe to eat, even though they continue to be highly unhealthy, processed slices of potatoes drenched with fat and salt."[23]

Organic foods seem to be another one of those food choices we worry about instead of changing the way we eat. "If you can afford them, buy them," recommends New York University professor Marion Nestle, PhD, MPH. "It really is a personal choice but how can anyone think substances, such as pesticides capable of killing insects, can be good for you?"[24]

But American Dietetic Association spokeswoman Keecha Harris says, "There is no evidence that organic foods are superior over traditional foods."[25]

People often cite health concerns to justify their opposition to pumping antibiotics and hormones into farm animals. The assumption that meat would be safe to eat if it didn't have antibiotics and hormones pumped into it is not very relevant. Long before modern chemicals were introduced into our food, people still began to experience more cancer and heart disease when they started to eat more animal-based foods.[26]

Michael Pollan writes in his book, *The Defense of Food*, that we should stick to real food and not edible food-like substances. He states that "...there is plenty of evidence that a person's health will improve with a simple shift in eating habits away from animal products and highly processed foods to plant products and 'real food'."[27]

You may feel better about eating an organic Oreo than a conventional Oreo, but organic junk food is still junk food.

One thing the experts agree on: Regardless of whether you choose locally grown, organic, or conventional foods, the important thing is to eat plenty of fruits and vegetables. The health benefits of such a diet far outweigh any potential risks from pesticide exposure.[28]

"Do you eat fish or take fish oil?"

In the November 2003 issue of the *Journal of Nutrition*, researcher Connie Stripp found that the risk of a woman developing breast cancer increased when she ate more fish. These findings are exactly the opposite of most of those found in experiments done on laboratory animals.[29]

Here are a few possible reasons:

> Fish and fish fat are known to suppress our cancer-fighting immune system.

> Fish is contaminated with cancer-causing

environmental chemicals like heavy metals and pesticides.

➢ Cooking fish produces powerful carcinogens called heterocyclic amines.[30]

According to Dr. John McDougall, "One of the reasons that fish has been touted as a health food is based on studies of long-lived peoples." At one time, the Japanese were healthy and lived longer than their American counterparts. Their diet contained some fish. However, at the time, they were healthy because of their starch-based diet of rice with added vegetables and only tiny amounts of fish.[31]

Unfortunately, many Japanese have started consuming a meat-based diet and their health concerns have become the same as those in the West.[32]

Doctors seem to be as misled as the rest of us, as they will encourage their patients with high cholesterol levels to get off of red meat and to start eating fish or chicken. But, fish and chicken are as high in cholesterol as beef or pork.[33]

"In studies that feed people fish oil, C-reactive protein levels (CRP) and other inflammatory markers don't budge," says Ishwarlal Jialal of the University of California, Davis Medical Center. [34] C-reactive protein is a substance in the blood produced by the liver and is an indicator of inflammation in the body. [35]

Researchers in Italy saw CRP and other inflammatory markers drop in people assigned to eat a Mediterranean diet. "They ate so many nice things—fruits, vegetables, nuts, whole grains," says Jialal.[36]

Eskimos have fatal nosebleeds because they eat so much fish. If we thin our blood too much with fish and omega-3s and aspirin, and we get into an automobile accident, we could bleed to death. If an artery in the brain were to rupture, such as occurs in a hemorrhagic stroke, you would want the blood to clot to stop the bleeding.[37]

Another reason not to eat fish or take fish oil capsules is because of the methyl mercury. This is one of the most toxic chemicals, and high levels in humans can cause heart attacks. Methyl mercury can also promote free radical formation as well as inflammation.[38]

In a recent *New York Times* story, Marian Burros writes, "Laboratory tests found so much mercury in tuna sushi from 20 Manhattan stores and restaurants that at most of them, a regular diet of six pieces a week would exceed the levels considered acceptable by the Environmental Protection Agency."[39]

Large doses of fish oil can increase the risk of hemorrhagic stroke, suppress the immune system, and decrease glucose control in people with diabetes.[40]

We need our immune system functioning at full capacity to fight off infections and cancer. Strengthening the immune system is a key strategy in cancer prevention and survival.[41]

The risk for developing melanoma is directly related to the degree to which the immune system is suppressed.[42]

Fatty foods can impair your immune cells' ability to

work. While many people avoid animal fats, they give themselves free rein with vegetable oils. But when it comes to boosting immunity, you want to minimize all fats and oils. This includes fish oils.[43]

Free oils, including fish oils, may be toxic to body tissues. Both omega-3 and omega-6 fats are associated with an increased risk of opacification of the lens of the eye, resulting in the formation of cataracts.[44]

Fish oil is very high in calories and can cause weight gain. People who don't lose weight on a plant-based diet, are probably still holding on to their oils. Many experts tout the benefits of a Mediterranean diet; and of course, if it is loaded with olive oil rather than fruits and vegetables, it will make you fat.[45]

Most importantly, worldwide population studies tell us that the lower the total fat intake, the less the risk of common cancers, such as breast, colon, and prostate.[46]

"Do you take supplements?"

Many people think they can replace the effects of a bad diet by adding supplements. Nutrition is a very complex biological system, so it doesn't make any sense to take isolated nutrient supplements.[47]

The supplement industry has grown much like the pharmaceutical industry, and there are huge profits to be made. Americans want to continue eating their customary foods and then they want to take a few supplements to make up for the lack of nutrients in them.[48]

Medical experts are becoming concerned that Americans are overdoing their vitamin consumption. As many as 70% of the population is taking supplements, convinced that the pills will make them healthier.[49]

But researchers say that multivitamins have not been shown to prevent any disease, and that it is easy to reach high enough doses of certain vitamins and minerals to actually increase the risk of disease.[50]

Dr. Benjamin Caballero, director of the Center for Human Nutrition at Johns Hopkins, does not take vitamins. "There is no disease I know of that is prevented by multivitamins," he says.[51]

Dr. Caballero also notes that large, rigorous studies that were supposed to show that individual vitamins prevented disease ended up showing the opposite. Those who took the vitamins actually had more of the disease it was meant to prevent.[52]

Two large randomized trials of vitamin A and beta-carotene that researchers hoped would show a protective value against cancer found no benefit, and one found that participants who took the supplements had more cancer.[53]

Dr. Caballero said people were deluding themselves if they thought multivitamins could make up for poor diets. "People are looking for the magic bullet. It does not exist."[54]

Antioxidants are very important, but only when they are consumed as food, not as supplements. Vitamin B_{12} is the only nutrient that we no longer get in our vegetables, since most of the soil is depleted of it.[55]

If you have not eaten any animal products for three years, or you are pregnant or breastfeeding, you should consider taking a small B_{12} supplement on occasion.[56]

"What if I have a family history of cancer?"

According to Dr. Campbell, "The bulk of resources in science and health during the past decade has shifted to genetic research. This might explain why some perfectly healthy young women have had their breasts removed simply because they were found to carry genes that are linked to cancer. All of this hoopla misses the point that not all genes are fully activated all the time and genes that are not activated are dormant. Dormant genes do not have any effect on our health."[57]

Even if we don't know exactly which risks we are predisposed to, we do know how to control those risks. Nutrition primarily determines whether the disease will ever do its damage. Rats that were given high doses of the aflatoxin, a known carcinogen, could become healthy, active, and cancer-free if they were fed low-protein diets.[58]

Breast cancer is thought to be initiated in adolescence and not become detectable until after menopause. Does this mean that these women should start smoking and eating more chicken-fried steak because they're doomed anyway? What do we do, given that many of us may already have an initiated chronic disease lurking in our bodies, waiting to explode decades from now?[59]

In humans, we have seen research findings showing that a whole-foods, plant-based diet reverses advanced heart disease, helps obese people lose weight, and helps diabetics get off their medication and return to a more normal, pre-diabetes life. Research has also shown that advanced melanoma, the deadly form of skin cancer, might be slowed down or reversed by lifestyle changes.[60]

Some diseases, of course, do appear to be irreversible. The autoimmune diseases seem most frightening because once the body turns against itself, it may become unstoppable. And yet, amazingly, even some of these diseases may be slowed by diet. Evidence shows that rheumatoid arthritis can be slowed by diet, as can multiple sclerosis.[61]

Dr. Campbell says, "The latest fads, the newest headlines, and the most recent study results are put into a useful context. We need not leap from our seats every time a chemical is called a carcinogen, every time a new diet book hits the shelf, or every time a headline screams about solving disease through genetic research."[62]

He continues: "The data from the China Study suggest that what we have come to consider as 'normal' illnesses of aging are really not normal. In fact, these findings indicate that the vast majority perhaps 80 to 90% of all cancers, cardiovascular diseases, and other forms of degenerative illness can be prevented, at least until very old age, simply by adopting a plant-based diet." [63]

"Are there any objective ways to determine if I'm on the right track?"

One of the easiest ways to give you a quick score as to how you are doing with your health is the new employee incentive cards offered by Whole Foods. These cards are based on the health scores of individual team members; the healthier they are, the bigger their discount on Whole Foods groceries and merchandise.[64]

By checking the chart below, if you worked at Whole Foods, which discount would your statistics allow you to get?[65]

Level	Discount	Nicotine	Blood Pressure	Cholesterol	BMI
Bronze	22%	NO	140/90	<195	<30
Silver	25%	NO	130/80	<180	<28
Gold	27%	NO	120/80	<165	<26
Platinum	30%	NO	110/70	<150	<24

Body Mass Index (BMI) is a number calculated from a person's weight and height, and is a reliable indicator of body fatness.[66]

Weight in relation to height	BMI Score
Underweight	<18.5
Normal weight	18.5 – 24.9
Overweight	25 – 29.9
Obese	30+

In population studies, the more that animal products were a part of the diet, the higher the BMI scores were.[67]

Population Group	Average BMI
Vegans	22
Vegetarians who consume milk and eggs	26.75
Vegetarians who eat fish	28
Vegetarians who eat meat once a week	29
Nonvegetarians	32

To lower your BMI scores, you will want to lower the fat content in your diet.[68]

Food	Fat Content (%/calories from fat)
Leanest beef	29%
Skinless chicken breast	23%
Sea trout	32%
White tuna	16%
Broccoli	8%
Beans	4%
Sweet potato	1%

Chapter 9:
A Ten-Day
"Getting Started"
Program

I am always doing that
which I can not do, in order that I may
learn how to do it.

~ Pablo Picasso

You will want to consider this a permanent change to your lifestyle, but I will get you started with this ten-day program. The recipes are basic and easy. As you get used to the program, you will want to branch out and try finding new recipes.

As you begin, let me encourage you not to simply dabble with dietary changes. Much as we might like to pretend that small dietary changes help, the fact is that trimming a little fat here and adding a piece of fruit there does very little.

If you are overweight, you will begin to lose weight. You could possibly lose between one and six pounds in these first five days. If you have suffered from chronic indigestion, you will notice that fading away as you continue to eat the plant-based diet. If you have severe angina pains or advanced atherosclerosis, you will be able to take walks without chest pains. Your blood cholesterol should begin to fall and your blood pressure will drop. At the end of the ten days, you'll actually feel healthier.

D A Y 1

And she won't eat oatmeal?
~ Dr. John McDougall

BREAKFAST

Cantaloupe / oatmeal*

*Oatmeal: Cook 5 minutes per package directions. Sprinkle with cinnamon or nutmeg. Add a little low-fat soy milk and raisins if you like.

LUNCH

Fast Pizza* / apple

*Fast Pizza: Separate 1 whole-wheat pita bread into circles. Spread each with tomato sauce. Sprinkle with basil, oregano, chopped onions, green peppers, mushrooms, and/or alfalfa sprouts. Bake at 350 degrees for 10 minutes.

DINNER

Asian Vegetable Salad** / Indian Rice Salad***/ pear

**Asian Vegetable Salad: In a large bowl, mix together 2 grated carrots, 10 halved cherry tomatoes, 1 chopped English cucumber, and 2 minced medium scallions. In a small jar, whisk together the dressing: 1 minced garlic clove, 1/4 tsp. red pepper flakes, 1 tsp. grated ginger root, 2 tbsp. rice wine vinegar, 1 tsp. red miso paste. Pour dressing over salad and refrigerate one hour before serving.

***Indian Rice Salad: Cook brown rice according to instructions. Cool and mix with raisins and cashews. Add the following non-irradiated spices for extra good health: turmeric, cumin, coriander.

EXERCISE

Walk 5 minutes in the morning and 10 minutes in the evening.

D
A
Y

2

If you want to eat bacon and eggs for breakfast and then take cholesterol-lowering medication, that's your right.

~ John Robbins, author

BREAKFAST

Brown rice (warmed from a previous meal) / sliced bananas / blueberries

LUNCH

Organic Sunshine Burger* with whole wheat bread, mustard, lettuce, sliced tomatoes, and sliced onions / banana

> ***Organic Sunshine Burgers** are made of sunflower seeds and grains, and can be found in the frozen food section of most health food stores.

DINNER

Whole wheat thin spaghetti and marinara sauce / tossed green salad

EXERCISE

Walk 5 minutes in the morning and 15 minutes in the evening.

D

A

Y

3

Eat food. Not too much. Mostly plants.
~ Michael Pollan

BREAKFAST

Hash Brown Potatoes* with barbecue sauce or salsa /
orange

*Hash Brown Potatoes: Look for frozen hash browns
that don't contain oil.

LUNCH

Quick Pasta Salad* / grapes

*Quick Pasta Salad: Cook 1 cup whole wheat or
spinach macaroni per package directions. Mix
cooked macaroni with chopped scallions, green
peppers, broccoli, celery, carrots, pimientos, and 1/4
cup low-sodium, oil-free salad dressing.

DINNER

American Vegetable Stew* / brown rice / apple

*American Vegetable Stew: Cook 2 cups vegetable
broth with 2 tbsp. chopped purple onion, 1 clove
minced garlic, 2 chopped potatoes, 1 chopped
carrot, 1 chopped celery stalk, 1 can tomatoes, and
1 can water. When vegetables are tender, blend in
blender until smooth. Put mixture back into soup
pot and add 1 can drained corn, 1 tbsp. parsley, 1/2
tsp. paprika, 1/2 tsp. basil, 1/2 tsp. chili powder, 1/4
tsp. dry mustard, 1/4 tsp. cumin, and 1/4 tsp. black
pepper. Heat and serve over cooked rice.

EXERCISE

Walk 10 minutes in the morning and 10 minutes in
the evening.

D

A

Y

4

If slaughterhouses had glass walls, we'd all be vegetarians.
~ Linda McCartney

BREAKFAST

Hot 7-grain cereal / peach slices

LUNCH

Baked potato / green salad / honeydew melon

DINNER

Bean and Rice Burritos* / tossed green salad

*Bean and Rice Burritos: Place 2 cans rinsed and drained pinto beans into saucepan and mash them with a potato masher. Add 1/2 cup cooked brown rice, 1 minced garlic clove, 1/4 tsp. chili powder, 1/4 tsp. cumin, and ¾ cup water; heat 5–10 minutes. Heat 6 whole wheat or corn tortillas in a preheated skillet just to soften. Place a line of bean mixture down the middle of each tortilla. Top with chopped lettuce, scallions, tomato, and salsa. Tuck the ends and roll into a burrito. Serve immediately.

EXERCISE

Walk 10 minutes in the morning and 15 minutes in the evening.

D

Cows' milk, by design, grows a 90-pound calf into a 2,000-pound cow over the course of two years.
~ The Skinny Bitch

A

BREAKFAST

Shredded Wheat or Grape-Nuts with frozen wild blueberries topped with cinnamon / rice cake with no-sugar raspberry or strawberry jam

Y

LUNCH

Warm whole wheat pita bread stuffed with kidney beans and veggies / banana

DINNER

5

Whole wheat thin spaghetti and Spinach Pesto Sauce* / Rice and Corn Salad**

*Spinach Pesto Sauce: Cook two bunches of spinach in small amount of water just until barely tender. Drain, reserving the liquid, and put the spinach in the blender with 2 cloves minced garlic, 1/4 cup chopped parsley, and 2 tbsp. fresh chopped basil. Blend until smooth, adding a little cooking liquid if necessary.

**Rice and Corn Salad: Mix 1 cup cooked brown rice, 1 cup thawed frozen corn, 1 chopped tomato, 1/4 cup chopped green pepper, 1/4 cup chopped green onions, and 1/4 cup finely chopped fresh parsley. Dressing: 1 tbsp. wine vinegar, 1 tbsp. water, 1 tbsp. soy sauce, 1/4 tsp. Dijon mustard, dash Tabasco sauce.

EXERCISE

Walk 15 minutes in the morning and 15 minutes in the evening.

D
A
Y
6

Simply adding milk to tea blocks any health benefits the tea might have.
~ The University of Berlin in the *European Heart Journal*

BREAKFAST

Grapefruit / hash brown potatoes with salsa

LUNCH

Quick Garbanzo Bean Soup* / sliced tomatoes

> ****Quick Garbanzo Bean Soup:** Sauté 1 small chopped onion, 1 cup minced fresh parsley, 2 large cloves pressed garlic, and 1 tsp. cumin in 1/4 cup water. Blend 3 cans garbanzo beans (undrained) in blender before adding to vegetable mixture along with 1/2 cup water, 1/4 cup freshly squeezed lemon juice, and a dash of cayenne pepper.

DINNER

Bulgur Chick Pea Salad* / assorted vegetable hors d'oeuvres / green beans

> ***Bulgur Chick Pea Salad:** Pour 2 cups boiling water over 1 cup bulgur wheat. Let stand one hour. In small bowl, beat together 1/4 cup olive oil, 1/2 cup lemon juice, and a dash of salt and pepper. Pour over bulgur and mix with fork. Place bulgur mixture in the bottom of a nice glass bowl and cover with layers of (in this order) 1 cup chopped green onion, 1 can garbanzo beans (drained), 1 cup chopped fresh parsley, and 1 cup grated carrots. Cover and refrigerate for one hour. Toss right before serving.

EXERCISE

Walk 20 minutes in the morning and 20 minutes in the evening.

D
A
Y

7

Just read the ingredients. If they are healthy, wholesome, and pure – dive in.
~ The Skinny Bitch

BREAKFAST

Multi-Mix Cold Cereal* with rice milk or low fat soy milk / sliced bananas

> ***Multi-Mix Cereal:** Combine 1/3 cup cooked brown rice, 1/3 cup quick-cooking oatmeal (uncooked), 1/3 cup Grape Nuts with cinnamon, raisins, and sliced banana.

LUNCH

Whole wheat pita bread stuffed with Hummus* and romaine lettuce / apple

> ***Hummus:** In a food processor blend 1 can drained garbanzo beans, 1/4 cup olive oil, 1 tbsp. lemon juice, 1 tsp. cumin. Add reserve liquid from beans if you need more liquid.

DINNER

Black Bean Soup* / Tomato Cucumber and Onion Salad with Vinegar / Cantaloupe

> ***Black Bean Soup:** Sauté in 1 tsp. olive oil: 1 chopped onion, 1 stalk celery, 2 carrots, and 4 cloves garlic for 3–4 minutes. Stir in 2 tbsp. chili powder, 1 tbsp. cumin, and a pinch of black pepper. Add 4 cups vegetable broth, 2 cans black beans, and 1 can corn. Meanwhile, in a blender, process 2 cans black beans with 1-14 oz. can crushed tomatoes. Stir into boiling soup mixture, reduce heat to low, and simmer for 15 minutes.

EXERCISE

Walk 20 minutes in the morning and 20 minutes in the evening.

D
A
Y

8

But there are still plenty of chickens out there with arsenic.

~ Marian Burros, New York Times

BREAKFAST:

Microwaved Baked Potato* with marinara sauce and sliced scallions

> ***Microwaved Baked Potato:** Puncture potatoes several times with a fork or small sharp knife. Place in a microwave-safe dish and cook on high for 7–8 minutes or until tender.

LUNCH:

Whole wheat pita pockets with white beans and vegetables

DINNER:

Quinoa with Sweet Potatoes and Mushrooms* / zucchini slices

> ***Quinoa with Sweet Potatoes and Mushrooms:** Stir 1/3 cup quinoa in a saucepan over medium heat until it begins to take on a toasty aroma; about 5 minutes. Pour in 1 cup water and 1/8 tsp. salt. Bring to a boil, then reduce heat to medium-low, cover, and simmer until the quinoa is tender; about 20 minutes.
>
> Meanwhile, heat 1 tsp. olive oil in a large skillet over medium heat. Stir in 2 cloves minced garlic and 1 small chopped onion, and cook until the onion has softened and turned translucent; about 5 minutes. Add 1 cup sliced mushrooms, 1 small sweet potato (peeled and diced), 1/4 tsp. cayenne pepper, and 1/2 tsp. black pepper. Cover the skillet, reduce heat to medium-low, and cook until the sweet potato is soft; about 20 minutes, stirring occasionally. Pour a splash of water into the skillet if needed to keep the vegetables from

burning. Spoon the vegetable mixture over a bed of quinoa, and sprinkle with 1/4 cup toasted, chopped pecans to serve.

EXERCISE

Walk 20 minutes in the morning and 20 minutes in the evening.

D

A

Y

9

If you want to get skinny, you can only rely on yourself.
~ The Skinny Bitch

BREAKFAST

Nutri-Grain cereal with low fat soy milk / apple slices

LUNCH

Warm corn tortilla topped with beans, tomatoes, lettuce, and salsa.

DINNER

Quinoa with Chick Peas and Tomatoes* / cauliflower florets**

> ***Quinoa with Chick Peas and Tomatoes:** Cook quinoa per package instructions. When done, stir in 1 can drained garbanzo beans, 1 chopped tomato, 1 clove minced garlic, 3 tbsp. lime juice, and 2 tsp. olive oil. Season with 1/2 tsp. cumin and a pinch of salt and pepper. Sprinkle with 1/2 tsp. chopped fresh parsley to serve.

> Cut ****cauliflower florets** in quarters and let sit for 5–10 minutes to allow time for the production of phenethyl isothiocyanates to form once cruciferous vegetables are cut. Then sprinkle them with turmeric and sauté on medium heat in a few tablespoons of vegetable broth for 5 minutes. Remove from the heat and drizzle a teaspoon of olive oil over the top. Season with sea salt and pepper to taste.

EXERCISE

Walk 20 minutes in the morning and 20 minutes in the evening.

DAY

10

The findings from the China Study indicate that the **lower** *the percentage of animal-based foods that are consumed, the* **greater** *the health benefits. So it's not unreasonable to assume that the optimum percentage of animal-based products is* **zero**, *at least for anyone with a predisposition for a degenerative disease.*

~ T. Colin Campbell, PhD

BREAKFAST

Grapefruit / breakfast quinoa with chopped apples, raisins, cinnamon, and soy or rice milk.

LUNCH

Peasant Salad* / french bread

*Peasant Salad: Chop two tomatoes, 1 cucumber, 1 yellow pepper and 1 small onion. Add 1/8 cup fresh chopped basil, 1 tbsp. capers, 1 minced garlic clove, and 1/2 cup oil-free Italian dressing.

DINNER

Black Beans* / rice / broiled tomatoes

*Black Beans: In large skillet, heat 1 tsp. olive oil. Cook 1 small chopped onion, 1 minced garlic clove, and 1/2 cup chopped green pepper until crisp tender; stir in 1 cup diced tomatoes, 1-15 oz. can drained black beans (drained, reserving liquid), and 1/2 tsp. thyme. Cook 3 minutes. Add 3 tbsp. cider vinegar, 1/2 tsp. hot pepper sauce, and the reserved bean liquid. Continue to cook 5 minutes. Serve over rice and garnish with lime wedge.

EXERCISE

Walk 30 minutes in the morning and 15 minutes in the evening (or vice versa, depending on your preference).

SNACKS

Snack on fruits, vegetables, instant soups, baked fat-free tortilla chips and salsa, pretzels, brown rice cakes, and whole grain crackers. Other snacks could include boiled red potatoes, canned garbanzo beans, popcorn, leftovers from last night's dinner, frozen juice popsicles, or sorbet.

EXERCISE

If you are already doing an exercise program that makes you feel good, continue it. Otherwise, you will want to walk, swim, or bicycle.

Eating Out

BEVERAGES

Order water—it is the ideal beverage. Non-caffeinated (herbal) teas are available in most restaurants, or can be brought from home as every restaurant can supply you with hot water.

RESTAURANT BREAKFAST IDEAS

▷ Hot Cereal: Order oatmeal, cream of wheat, polenta, or corn grits (without butter, cream, or milk).

▷ Cold Cereal: Most restaurants have Shredded Wheat, Nutri-Grain, or Grape-Nuts (top them with hot water, cold apple juice, or bring along low-fat soy milk). You can also just add fruit and eat the cereal dry.

▷ Other: Hash browns; whole wheat toast, dry with a no-sugar fruit jam or a tiny bit of honey.

Restaurant Lunches and Dinners

▷ Baked Potatoes: You can eat one or two, as they are less than 150 calories each. Eat them plain or sprinkled with chives, onions, vegetable seasoning, lemon juice and/or vinegar or salsa.

▷ Salad Bars: Look closely to find the vegetables that are not covered in sauces or oils. Use lemon juice or vinegar for your dressing.

▷ Sandwiches: Ask for a sandwich on whole grain bread with lettuce, bean sprouts, tomatoes, onions, green peppers, and any other low fat vegetables.

▷ Steamed Vegetables: Sprinkled with lemon juice or vinegar.

▷ Beans: You can ask for a bowl of beans.

▷ Breads: Pita breads, corn tortillas.

▷ Pizza: Whole wheat crust with marinara sauce and onions, green pepper, mushrooms, and/or tomatoes. Pineapple chunks are good on vegetarian pizzas, too. Ask them to leave off the cheese.

▷ Chinese: Ask for whole grain rice with tofu and vegetables.

▷ Japanese: Miso soup and a cucumber and carrot salad.

▷ Greek: Pita bread with hummus and tabouleh.

▷ Thai: Green papaya and cabbage salad or sweet and sour vegetables over brown rice.

▷ Indian: Ask the chef to prepare you a vegetarian meal without added oil and dairy products.

Invitations to Parties

Eat something healthy before you go so you won't be tempted by the foods which are not appropriate for your lifestyle.

Losing Too Much Weight?

Eat more whole-grain bread and dried fruits. If you need more, you can eat moderate amounts of avocados, nuts, peanut butter, olives, and tofu.

Not Losing Enough Weight?

Stay away from breads. Limit fruits to three a day. Concentrate on green and yellow vegetables, and don't forget to exercise. Limit your alcoholic beverages to one a day and make sure you have eliminated carbonated drinks. Be sure you have weaned yourself off of oils, nuts, avocados, and olives.

Do You Have Indigestion?

Try cutting back on raw onions, cucumbers, radishes, salsas, and green and red peppers. Also, you will want to make sure you have eliminated coffee, alcohol, and carbonated drinks.

Some Challenges You May Face

When you decide to transition to a plant-based diet, you may encounter some challenges such as:

- Stomach upset as your digestive system adjusts
- More time involved as you learn new recipes and discover new restaurants.

> ❧ You'll need to adjust psychologically. No matter how full the plate is, you were trained that a meal is not complete without meat.

> ❧ You may not be able to go to the same restaurants you used to go to and you will need to adjust your ordering.

> ❧ Your friends, family and colleagues may not be supportive. Many people may seem to find it threatening that you are now a vegan.

REMEMBER THE FOUR NEW FOOD GROUPS: VEGETABLES, WHOLE GRAINS, FRUIT, LEGUMES

The ability of nutrition to prevent the occurrence of cancer is now beyond dispute. In fact, cancer rates were reduced 50% in the people who ate the most fruits and vegetables, with the greatest reduction being in cancers of the esophagus, oral cavity, larynx, pancreas, stomach, colon, rectum, bladder, cervix, ovary, endometrium, prostate, and breast.

I wish you the very best of luck as you transition into your new life.

Bibliography

Becoming vegan was probably
the most profound change I have
ever made in my life.

~ Kathy Freston

Agence France-Presse (AFP). "Green Tea, Mushrooms Combat Cancer." *Bangkok Post*, March 18, 2009. http://www.bangkokpost.com/breakingnews/137800/green-tea-mushrooms-combat-cancer (accessed March 2010).

———. "Red Wine and Dark Chocolate Cancer Killers: Researcher." *Physorg*, February 11, 2010. http://www.physorg.com/news185087626.html (accessed April 2010).

———. "Researchers Back Cancer-Fighting Properties of Papaya." *Vancouver Sun*, March 9, 2010. http://www.vancouversun.com/story_print.html?id=2662932&sponsor (accessed March 2010).

———. "Sugary Soft Drinks Linked to Pancreatic Cancer." *Bangkok Post*, Feb. 9, 2010. http://www.bangkokpost.com/news/health/167914/sugary-soft-drinks-linked-to-pancreatic-cancer-study (accessed March 2010).

American Cancer Society. "Can Cancer be Prevented?" http://our.cancer.org/docroot/CRI/content/CRI_2_4_2x_Can_cancer_be_prevented.asp (accessed March 2010).

———. "Chronic Inflammation Linked to Cancer." http://our.cancer.org/docroot/NWS/content/NWS_1_1x_Chronic_Inflammation_Linked_to_Cancer.asp (accessed April 2010).

———. "Common Questions about Diet and Cancer." http://our.cancer.org/docroot/PED/content/PED_3_2X_Common_Questions_About_Diet_and_Cancer.asp (accessed April 2010).

———. "Nine Risk Factors Account for One-third of World's Cancer Deaths." http://our.cancer.org/docroot/NWS/content/NWS_2_1x_Nine_Risk_Factors_Account_for_One-Third_of_Worlds_Cancer_Deaths.asp (accessed April 2010).

———. "Oncogenes and Tumor Suppressor Genes." http://our.cancer.org/docroot/eto/content/eto_1_4x_oncogenes_and_tumor_suppressor_genes.asp (accessed April 2010).

———. "Tobacco-Related Cancers Fact Sheet." http://our.cancer.org/docroot/PED/content/PED_10_2x_Tobacco-Related_Cancers_Fact_Sheet.asp?sitearea=PED (accessed March 2010).

———. "What Are the Key Statistics for Breast Cancer?" http://our.cancer.org/docroot/cri/content/cri_2_4_1x_what_are_the_key_statistics_for_breast_cancer_5.asp (accessed April 2010).

———. "What Are the Risk Factors for Cervical Cancer?" http://our.

cancer.org/docroot/cri/content/cri_2_4_2X_what_are_the_risk_
factors_for_cervical_cancer_8.asp (accessed April 2010).

————. "What Are the Risk Factors for Gallbladder Cancer?" http://our.
cancer.org/docroot/CRI/content/CRI_2_4_2X_What_are_the_risk_
factors_for_gall_bladder_cancer_68.asp (accessed April 2010).

————. "What Are the Risk Factors for Laryngeal and Hypopharyngeal
Cancers?" http://our.cancer.org/docroot/CRI/content/CRI_2_4_2X_
What_are_the_risk_factors_for_laryngeal_and_hypopharyngeal_
bladder_cancer_23.asp.

————. "What Causes Hodgkin Disease?" http://our.cancer.org/docroot/
CRI/content/CRI_2_2_2X_What_causes_Hodgkins_disease_Can_it_
be_prevented_20.asp (accessed April 2010).

American Heart Association. "What Your Cholesterol Levels Mean."
http://www.americanheart.org/presenter.jhtml?identifier=183
(accessed March 2010).

"Anesthesia May Affect Metastasis Risk after Cancer Surgery." Journal
of Anaesthesiology Clinical Pharmacology online report. http://www.
joacp.org/index.php?option=com_content&view=article&id=60&cat
id=1 (accessed April 2010).

Babayode, Christopher. "Wave Your Health Good-bye with Sky High
WiFi." WEEP News, August 28, 2009. http://weepnews.blogspot.
com/2009/08/thyroid-cancer-increase-puzzles-experts.html (accessed
May 2010).

Balbi, J. C., M. T. Larrinaga, E. De Stefani, M. Mendilaharsu, A. L.
Ronco, P. Boffetta, and P. Brennan. "Foods and Risk of Bladder
Cancer: A Case-control Study in Uruguay." European Journal of
Cancer Prevention 10, no. 5 (October 2001). http://www.ncbi.nlm.nih.
gov/pubmed/11711760 (accessed April 2010).

Ban Trans Fat. "About Trans Fat." http://www.bantransfats.com/
abouttransfat.html (accessed March 2010).

Barnard, Neal D. "A Plant-based Diet for Type-2 Diabetes." McDougall
Advanced Lecture Series, Santa Rosa, CA, February 20, 2010.

————. "Breaking the Food Seduction." McDougall Advanced Lecture
Series, Santa Rosa, CA, February 19, 2010.

————. Foods That Fight Pain: Revolutionary New Strategies for Maximum
Pain Relief. New York: Three Rivers Press, 1998.

Barnard, Neal D. and Reilly, Jennifer K. The Cancer Survivor's Guide:
Foods that help you fight back. Summertown, TN: Healthy Living

Publications, 2008.

Barrow, Karen. "The Link between Rheumatoid Arthritis and Lymphoma." Science*Daily*, November 17, 2009. http://sciencedaily. healthology.com/arthritis/article3960.htm (accessed April 2010).

Begley, Sharon. "We Fought Cancer... and Cancer Won." *Newsweek*, September 6, 2008. http://www.newsweek.com/2008/09/05/we-fought-cancer-and-cancer-won.html (accessed March 2010).

BioInfoBank Library. "Molecular Pathology of Cancer Cell." http:// lib. bioinfo.pl/courses/view/158 (accessed April 2010).

Bittman, Mark. "Eating Food That's Better for You, Organic or Not," *New York Times Week in Review*, March 21, 2009. http://www.nytimes. com/2009/03/22/weekinreview/22bittman.html (accessed April 2010).

Blaylock, Russell L. *Natural Strategies for Cancer Patients.* New York: Twin Streams/Kensington, 2003.

Brazma, Alvis, Helen Parkinson, Thomas Schlitt, and Mohammadreza Shojatalab. "A Quick Introduction to Elements of Biology - Cells, Molecules, Genes, Functional Genomics, Microarrays." European Bioinformatics Institute, October 2001. http://www.ebi.ac.uk/ microarray/biology_intro.html (accessed March 2010).

Brewer, George J. "Risks of Copper and Iron Toxicity during Aging in Humans." *Chemical Research in Toxicology* 23, no. 2 (December 7, 2009). http://pubs.acs.org/doi/abs/10.1021/tx900338d (accessed March 2010).

Brody, Jane E. "Huge Study of Diet Indicts Fat and Meat." *New York Times Science*, May 8, 1990. http://www.nytimes.com/1990/05/08/ science/huge-study-of-diet-indicts-fat-and-meat.html?pagewanted=1 (accessed March 2010).

Burros, Marian. "High Mercury Levels Are Found in Tuna Sushi." *New York Times Dining & Wine*, January 23, 2008. http://www.nytimes. com/2008/01/23/dining/23sushi.html (accessed February 2010).

Campbell, T. Colin. "Hidden Hazards of Animal Protein." McDougall Advanced Lecture Series DVD, Produced by John and Mary McDougall, 2008.

Campbell, T. Colin, and Thomas M. Campbell II. *The China Study: Startling Implications for Diet, Weight Loss and Long-term Health.* Dallas, TX: BenBella Books, 2006.

Cancer Prevention Coalition. "International Scientific Committee Warns of Serious Risks of Breast and Prostate Cancer from Monsanto's

Hormonal Milk." http://www.preventcancer.com/press/releases/ march21_99.htm (accessed March 2010).

Cancer Project, The. "Ask the Expert - Eggs." http://www.cancerproject. org/ask/eggs.php (accessed April 2010).

———. "Diet and Cancer Research - Iron: the Double-Edged Sword." http://www.cancerproject.org/diet_cancer/nutrition/iron.php (accessed March 2010).

Cancer Research UK. "Pancreatic Cancer Risks and Causes." http:// www.cancerhelp.org.uk/type/pancreatic-cancer/about/pancreatic-cancer-risks-and-causes (accessed July 2010).

———. "What Causes Cancer?" http://www.cancerhelp.org.uk/about-cancer/causes-symptoms/causes/what-causes-cancer (accessed April 2010).

Centers for Disease Control and Prevention. "Body Mass Index." http:// www.cdc.gov/healthyweight/assessing/bmi/ (accessed April 2010).

———. "Lung Cancer Risk Factors." http://www.cdc.gov/cancer/lung/ basic_info/risk_factors.htm (accessed April 2010).

Challem, Jack. "Beating Breast Cancer: If Genes Don't Matter, What Does?" *Nutrition Reporter*, 2000. http://www.thenutritionreporter.com/ beating_breast_cancer.html (accessed March 2010).

Chan, June M., Meir J. Stampfer, Jing Ma, Peter H. Gann, J. Michael Gaziano, and Edward L. Giovannucci. "Dairy Products, Calcium, and Prostate Cancer Risk in the Physicians' Health Study." *American Journal of Clinical Nutrition* 74, no. 4 (October 2001), 549–554. http:// www.ajcn.org/cgi/content/full/74/4/549 (accessed March 2010).

Cheng, Maria. "Losing Breast Not Always Best for Cancer Patients." *Chicago Defender Online*, March 31, 2010. http://www. chicagodefender.com/article-7488-losing-breast-not-al.html (accessed April 2010).

CitySpur. "How to Prevent Cancer—A Detailed Study." Long Beach 10 Web site, from an article posted on Meditrendz (http://www. meditrendz.com/archives/2009/how-to-prevent-cancer-a-detailed-study/), March 11, 2009. http://longbeach10.cityspur.com/2009/11/23/ how-to-prevent-cancer-a-detailed-study/ (accessed March 2010).

Cohen, Robert. "Who Gets Bone Disease?" http://www.sunfood.net/ milk-bones.html (accessed April 2010).

Collins, Anne. "Protein and Diet Information." http://www.annecollins.

com/protein-diet.htm (accessed April 2010).

Conlin, Michelle. "Cellphones Cause Brain Tumors, Says New Report by International EMF Collaborative." *Bloomberg Businessweek*, August 26, 2009. http://www.businessweek.com/careers/managementiq/archives/2009/08/cellphones_caus.html (accessed April 2010).

Consumers Union. "Concern Over Canned Foods." *Consumer Reports*, December 2009. http://www.consumerreports.org/cro/magazine-archive/december-2009/food/bpa/overview/bisphenol-a-ov.htm (accessed April 2010).

———. "Risk Factors for Pancreas Cancer." *Consumer Reports: Health*. http://www.consumerreports.org/health/conditions-and-treatments/pancreas-cancer/what-is-it/risk-factors.htm (accessed June 6, 2010).

Crosta, Peter. "What Is Cancer? What Causes Cancer?" *Medical News Today*, n.d. http://www.medicalnewstoday.com/info/cancer-oncology/whatiscancer.php (accessed April 2010).

Daily Mail Staff Reporter. "Eating Tofu Can Slash Ovarian Cancer Risk." *Mail Online*, January 12, 2007. http://www.dailymail.co.uk/news/article-428478/Eating-tofu-slash-ovarian-cancer-risk.html (accessed April 2010).

Dana-Farber Cancer Institute. "Cancer Prevention Quick Facts" (sidebar on "February: National Cancer Prevention Month" page). http://www.dana-farber.org/can/monthly-cancer-awareness/national-cancer-prevention-month/ (accessed April 2010).

DNA Direct. "Who Is At Risk for Ovarian Cancer?" http://www.dnadirect.com/web/article/testing-for-genetic-disorders/breast-and-ovarian-cancer-risk/93/who-is-at-risk-for-ovarian-cancer (accessed April 2010).

Dotinga, Randy. "Meat Lovers Face Greater Risk of Bladder Cancer." *Bloomberg Businessweek*, April 20, 2010. http://www.businessweek.com/lifestyle/content/healthday/638268.html (accessed April 2010).

Dunaif, G. E., and T. C. Campbell. "Relative Contribution of Dietary Protein Level and Aflatoxin B1 Dose in Generation of Presumptive Preneoplastic Foci in Rat Liver." *Journal of the National Cancer Institute* 78, no. 2 (February 1987): 365–369.

Ellis-Christensen, Tricia. "What is Carrageenan?" Wisegeek.com, n.d. http://www.wisegeek.com/what-is-carrageenan.htm (accessed April 2010).

Farlow, Christine H. "Do You Eat Food with Any of These 9 Cancer-

Causing Chemicals?" *Healthy Eating Advisor*, 2004. http://www. healthyeatingadvisor.com/9cancer-causingchemicals.html (accessed March 2010).

Fayed, Lisa. "The Causes and Risk Factors of Cancer," About.com: Cancer, August 2006. http://cancer.about.com/od/causes/a/causesrisks. htm (accessed March 2010).

Freedman, Rory and Kim Barnouin. *Skinny Bitch: A No-Nonsense, Tough-Love Guide for Savvy Girls Who Want to Stop Eating Crap and Start Looking Fabulous!* Philadelphia: Running Press, 2005.

Freston, Kathy. *Quantum Wellness: A Practical and Spiritual Guide to Health and Happiness*. New York: Weinstein, 2008.

Frias, Claudia. "Oral Sex Linked to Increased Cancer Rates in Young People." *TerraUSA*, April 16, 2010. http://en.terra.com/dating-relationships/news/oral_sex_linked_to_increased_cancer_rates_in_young_people/hof9149 (accessed April 2010).

Gansler, Douglas. "A Deadly Ingredient in a Chicken Dinner." *Washington Post*, June 26, 2009. http://www.washingtonpost.com/wp-dyn/content/article/2009/06/25/AR2009062503381.html (accessed April 2010).

Good Housekeeping staff. "About the Anti-Aging Diet." *Good Housekeeping Diet and Health*, 2010. http://www.goodhousekeeping. com/health/diet/about-anti-aging-diet (accessed April 2010).

Gori, Gio B. "Diet and Nutrition in Cancer Causation." *Nutrition and Cancer: An International Journal* 1, no. 1 (Fall 1978): 5–8.

Hamblen, Matt. "Cell Phone, Cancer Link Claimed." *PC World*, August 29, 2009. http://www.pcworld.com/article/171012/cell_phone_cancer_link_claimed.html (accessed May 2010).

HealthCheck Systems. "Understanding Free Radicals and Antioxidants." http://www.healthchecksystems.com/antioxid.htm (accessed April 2010).

Healthcommunities.com. "Overview, Types of Bladder Cancer, Incidence." June 15, 1998. http://www.urologychannel.com/bladdercancer/index.shtml (accessed April 2010).

———. "Pancreatic Cancer Risk Factors." August 15, 1999. http://www. oncologychannel.com/pancreaticcancer/risk-factors.shtml (accessed April 2010).

Houben, M. P. W. A., W. J. Louwman, C. C. Tijssen, J. L. J. M. Teepen,

C. M. van Duijn, and J. W. W. Coebergh. "Hypertension as a Risk Factor for Glioma? Evidence from a Population-based Study of Comorbidity in Glioma Patients." *Oxford Journal: Annals of Oncology* 15, no. 8 (2004). http://annonc.oxfordjournals.org/content/15/8/1256. abstract (accessed April 2010).

Jemal, Ahmedin, Rebecca Siegel, Elizabeth Ward, Yongping Hao, Jiaquan Xu, Taylor Murray, and Michael J. Thun. "Cancer Statistics, 2008." *A Cancer Journal for Clinicians* 58 (February 20, 2008), 71–96. http://caonline.amcancersoc.org/cgi/content/full/58/2/71 (accessed April 2010).

Jones, Desiree. "Life Extension Daily News - Whole Grains Reduce Heart Disease 30 Percent, Diabetes in Women." Gibson's Healthful Living Blog, August 19, 2009. http://www.gibsonshealth.com/blog/?p=81 (accessed April 2010).

Kolata, Gina. "Vitamins: More May Be Too Many." *New York Times Science*, April 29, 2003. http://www.nytimes.com/2003/04/29/science/vitamins-more-may-be-too-many.html?pagewanted=1 (accessed April 2010).

Krulwich, Robert. "Bacteria Outnumber Cells in Human Body." National Public Radio Web site, July 1, 2006. http://www.npr.org/templates/story/story.php?storyId=5527426 (accessed March 2010).

Kulze, Ann. "Dr. Ann's 10-Steps to Prevent Breast Cancer." About. com Women's Health, last updated October 30, 2009. http://womenshealth.about.com/od/cancerprevention/a/10stepsprevbcan.htm (accessed April 2010).

Kushi, Lawrence H., P. J. Mink, A. R. Folsom, K. E. Anderson, W. Zheng, D. Lazovich, and T. A. Sellers. "Prospective Study of Diet and Ovarian Cancer." *American Journal of Epidemiology* 149, no. 1 (January 1, 1999). http://www.ncbi.nlm.nih.gov/pubmed/9883790 (accessed April 2010).

Kushi, Lawrence H., Tim Byers, Colleen Doyle, Elisa V. Bandera, Marji McCullough, Ted Gansler, Kimberly S. Andrews, Michael J. Thun, and The American Cancer Society 2006 Nutrition and Physical Activity Guidelines Advisory Committee. "American Cancer Society Guidelines on Nutrition and Physical Activity for Cancer Prevention." *CA: A Cancer Journal for Clinicians* 56 (September–October 2006):254-281. http://caonline.amcancersoc.org/cgi/content/full/56/5/254 (accessed February 2010).

Leaf, Clifton. "Why We're Losing the War on Cancer." *Fortune*, March 22, 2004. http://money.cnn.com/magazines/fortune/fortune_archive/2004/03/22/365076/index.htm.

Leukemia & Lymphoma Society. "Facts and Statistics." July 1, 2009. http://www.leukemia-lymphoma.org/all_page?item_id=12486 (accessed April 2010).

Liebman, Bonnie. "Slow Burn: How Inflammation Can Trigger a Heart Attack." The Free Library (originally published in *Nutrition Action Healthletter*, January 1, 2009). http://www.thefreelibrary.com/Slow+burn:+how+inflammation+can+trigger+a+heart+attack.-a0192898839 (accessed April 2010).

Life Extension. "Health Concerns: Leukemia." http://www.lef.org/protocols/cancer/leukemia_01.htm (accessed April 2010).

Lijinsky, W. "N-Nitroso Compounds in the Diet." *Mutation Research* 443, no. 1-2 (July 15, 1999). http://www.ncbi.nlm.nih.gov/pubmed/10415436 (accessed April 2010).

Mackey, John. "Whole Foods Markets' Efforts to Change the World through Better Nutrition." Presentation, McDougall Advanced Study Lecture Series, Santa Rosa, CA, February 19, 2010.

Mahler, Mike. "Getting Big and Strong on a Vegan Diet." Bodybuilding, n.d. http://www.bodybuilding.com/fun/mahler53.htm (accessed March 2010).

———. "Making the Vegan Diet Work." Mahler's Aggressive Strength Nutrition Articles, n.d. http:// www.mikemahler.com/articles/vegan_diet.html (accessed March 2010).

Mangels, Reed. "Protein in the Vegan Diet." The Vegetarian Resource Group (originally published in *Simply Vegan: Quick Vegetarian Meals* by Debra Wasserman and Reed Mangels). http://www.vrg.org/nutrition/protein.htm (accessed April 2010).

Mayo Clinic staff. "Cancer Prevention: Seven Steps to Reduce Your Risk." Mayo Clinic Adult Health, n.d. http://www.mayoclinic.com/health/cancer-prevention/CA00024 (accessed April 2010).

McDougall, John. "A Starch-based Diet Supports Spontaneous Healing: Atherosclerosis, Arthritis, and Sometimes Cancer." *McDougall Newsletter*, May 2009. http://www.drmcdougall.com/misc/2009nl/may/090500.pdf (accessed April 2010).

———. "Acrylamide Poisoning: Cancer from Overcooked

Carbohydrates?" *McDougall Newsletter*, June 2005. http://www. drmcdougall.com/misc/2005nl/june/050600acrylamide.htm (accessed May 2010).

———. "Dr. McDougall Disputes Major Medical Treatments." DVD, 2007, John McDougall.

———. "Dr. McDougall's Common Sense Nutrition." DVD, 2008 John McDougall.

———. "Favorite Five Articles from Recent Medical Journals." *McDougall Newsletter*, March 2010. http://www.drmcdougall.com/ misc/2010nl/mar/fav5.htm (accessed April 1, 2010).

———. "Low Vitamin D: One Sign of Sunlight Deficiency." *McDougall Newsletter*, September 2007. http://www.drmcdougall.com/misc/2007nl/ sep/070900.pdf (accessed April 2010).

———. "My Favorite Five Articles from Last Month's Medical Journals." *McDougall Newsletter*, December 2003. http://www. nealhendrickson.com/mcdougall/031200pufavorite5.htm (accessed March 2010).

———. "New Trans-Fat Labels: Too Little, Too Late." Dr. McDougall's Health and Medical Center Web site. http://www.drmcdougall.com/ res_trans_fat_labels.html (accessed April 2010).

———. "Salt: The Scapegoat for the Western Diet." *McDougall Newsletter*, August 2008. http://www.drmcdougall.com/misc/2008nl/ aug/salt.htm (accessed March 2010).

———. "Soy — Food, Wonder Drug, or Poison?" *McDougall Newsletter*, April 2005. http://www.drmcdougall.com/misc/2005nl/ april/050400pusoy.htm (accessed February 2010).

———. "Sunny Days, Keeping Those Clouds Away…" *McDougall Newsletter*, May 2005. http://www.drmcdougall.com/misc/pdf/ pdf050500nl.pdf (accessed March 2010).

———. "The Fallacy of Early Detection." Keynote Address: *McDougall Advanced Study Lecture Series,* Santa Rosa, CA, February 20, 2010.

———. "Vegan Diet Damages Baby's Brain – Sensationalism! People Love to Hear Good News about their Bad Habits!" *McDougall Newsletter*, February 2003. http://www.nealhendrickson.com/McDouga ll/030200puVeganDietDamages.htm (accessed March 2010).

———. "Vitamin D Pills Are of Little or No Benefit and Some Harm. So What to Do Now?" *McDougall Newsletter,* March 2010. http://www.

drmcdougall.com/misc/2010nl/mar/vitd.htm (accessed April 2010).

———. "When Friends Ask: Why Do You Avoid Adding Vegetable Oils?" *McDougall Newsletter*, August 2007. http://www.drmcdougall. com/misc/2007nl/aug/oils.htm (accessed February 2010).

McLean, Rob. "Milk – Calcium – Protein: Do They Protect from Osteoporosis?" Cyberparent.com. http://www.cyberparent.com/ nutrition/osteoporosiscausemilk.htm (accessed April 2010).

Medical News Today. "Multiple Dental X-Rays Raise Risk of Thyroid Cancer." http://www.medicalnewstoday.com/articles/191025.php (accessed July 2010).

MedicineNet.com. "Hodgkin's Disease Adult." http://www.medicinenet. com/hodgkins_disease/article.htm (accessed April 2010).

———. "Non-Hodgkin's Lymphoma (cont.)." http://www.medicinenet. com/non-hodgkins_lymphomas/page2.htm (accessed April 2010).

Medicineworld.org. "What Causes Cancer?" http://medicineworld.org/ cancer/page14.html (accessed April 2010).

Medline Plus Encyclopedia., "Brain Tumor – Primary – Adults." http:// www.nlm.nih.gov/medlineplus/ency/article/007222.htm (accessed April 2010).

———. "Endometrial Cancer." http://www.nlm.nih.gov/medlineplus/ ency/article/000910.htm (accessed April 2010).

———. "Schistosomiasis." http://www.nlm.nih.gov/medlineplus/ency/ article/001321.htm (accessed April 2010).

Melanoma Center. "Risk Factors: Suppressed Immune System." http:// www.melanomacenter.org/risk/sis.html (accessed March 2010).

Menon, Anjum, Sara Godward, et. al. "Dental X-rays and the Risk of Thyroid Cancer: A Case-control Study," *Acta Oncologica*, 49, no. 4 (May 2010): 447–453.

Miller, Maria. "Omega-3 Fats and Intelligence." Home School Math, n.d. http://www.homeschoolmath.net/teaching/fats-intelligence.php (accessed April 2010).

Morgan, L. Lloyd, Elizabeth Barris, Janet Newton, Eileen O'Connor, Alasdair Philips, Graham Philips, Camilla Rees, and Brian Stein. "Cellphones and Brain Tumors: Fifteen Reasons for Concern." *Radiation Research*, August 25, 2009. http://www.radiationresearch. org/pdfs/reasons_us.pdf (accessed March 2010).

Mouth Cancer Foundation. "Reduce Your Chances of Getting These Cancers." http://www.rdoc.org.uk/ (accessed April 2010).

National Cancer Institute. "Acrylamide in Food and Cancer Risk." http://www.cancer.gov/cancertopics/factsheet/risk/acrylamide-in-food (accessed April 2010).

———. "Alcohol and Breast Cancer Risk: New Findings." http://www. cancer.gov/cancertopics/causes/breast/alcoholuse0408 (accessed April 2010).

———. "Artificial Sweeteners and Cancer." http://www.cancer.gov/ cancertopics/factsheet/Risk/artificial-sweeteners (accessed April 2010).

———. "BRCA1 and BRCA2: Cancer Risk and Genetic Testing." http:// www.cancer.gov/cancertopics/factsheet/Risk/BRCA (accessed April 2010).

———. "Dioxins." Cancer Trends Progress Report — 2009–2010 Update. http://progressreport.cancer.gov/doc_detail.asp?pid=1&did= 2009&chid=91&coid=914&mid= (accessed April 2010).

———. "Fluoridated Water: Questions and Answers." http://www. cancer.gov/cancertopics/factsheet/Risk/fluoridated-water (accessed April 2010).

———. "Heterocyclic Amines in Cooked Meats." http://www.cancer. gov/cancertopics/factsheet/Risk/heterocyclic-amines (accessed April 2010).

———. "HIV Infection and Cancer Risk." http://www.cancer.gov/ cancertopics/factsheet/risk/hiv-infection (accessed April 2010).

———. "H. pylori and Cancer: Fact Sheet." http://www.cancer.gov/ cancertopics/factsheet/risk/h-pylori-cancer (accessed April 2010).

———. "Obesity and Cancer: Questions and Answers." http://www. cancer.gov/cancertopics/factsheet/Risk/obesity (accessed April 2010).

———. "Pesticides." Cancer Trends Progress Report — 2009-2010 Update. http://progressreport.cancer.gov/doc_detail.asp?pid=1&did= 2009&chid=91&coid=913&mid= (accessed April 2010).

———. "SEER Stat Fact Sheets: All Sites." Surveillance Epidemiology and End Results (SEER). http://seer.cancer.gov/statfacts/html/all.html (accessed April 2010).

National Health Service. "Mouth Cancer: Are You at Risk?" http:// www.nhs.uk/Livewell/cancer/Pages/Mouthcancer.aspx (accessed April 2010).

National Institutes of Health. "Teacher's Guide: Understanding Cancer." http://science-education.nih.gov/supplements/nih1/Cancer/guide/understanding2.htm (accessed April 2010).

———. "Understanding Cancer Series: Cancer." http://www.cancer.gov/cancertopics/understandingcancer/cancer/allpages (accessed April 2010).

National Research Council, Committee on Diet and Health. *Diet and Health: Implications for Reducing Chronic Disease Risk.* Washington, D.C.: National Academies Press, 1989. http://books.nap.edu/openbook.php?record_id=1222&page=599 (accessed April 2010).

Nelson, Nancy J. "Nurses' Health Study: Nurses Helping Science and Themselves." *Journal of the National Cancer Institute*, 92, no. 8, (April 19, 2000): 597–599. http://jnci.oxfordjournals.org/cgi/content/full/92/8/597 (accessed June 6, 2010).

Newcomb-Fernandez, Jennifer. "Cancer in the HIV-Infected Population." The Center for AIDS, Summer 2003. http://www.thebody.com/content/art16834.html (accessed April 2010).

New Jersey Department of Health and Senior Services. "Cancer Risk Factors." http://www.state.nj.us/health/cancer/cariskfactorsfsfinal02.htm (accessed April 2010).

New York Times Health Guide, "Physical Activity: Exercise's Effects on Other Conditions." *New York Times,* March 1, 2009. http://health.nytimes.com/health/guides/specialtopic/physical-activity/exercise's-effects-on-other-conditions.html (accessed April 2010).

NutritionMD. "Making Sense of Foods: Understanding the Problems with Dairy Products." http://www.nutritionmd.org/nutrition_tips/nutrition_tips_understand_foods/dairy.html (accessed April 2010).

Nutritional Supplements. "Essential Amino Acids." http://www.glisonline.com/essential-amino-acids.html (accessed April 2010).

Oransky, Ivan. "Sir Richard Doll." *The Lancet* 366, no. 9434 (August 6, 2005). http://www.thelancet.com/journals/lancet/article/PIIS0140-6736(05)67047-X/fulltext (accessed February 2010).

Pickart, Loren. "The Chemical Sunscreen Health Disaster." http://www.skinbiology.com/toxicsunscreens.html (accessed May 2010).

Pritikin Longevity Center and Spa. "Nathan Pritikin: Founder, The Pritikin Program." http://www.pritikin.com/index.php?option=com_content&view=article&id=61&Itemid=89 (accessed May 2010).

Pulde, Alona, and Matthew Lederman. *Keep It Simple, Keep It Whole: Your Guide to Optimum Health.* USA: Exsalus Health & Wellness Center, 2009.

Qadeer, M. A., N. Colabianchi, and M. F. Vaezi. "Is GERD a Risk Factor for Laryngeal Cancer?" *Laryngoscope* 115, no. 3 (March 2005). http://www.ncbi.nlm.nih.gov/pubmed/15744163 (accessed April 2010).

ReadersDigest.com. "Top 10 Antioxidant-Rich Fruits and Veggies." http://www.rd.com/living-healthy/top-10-antioxidant-rich-fruits-and-veggies/article16245.html (accessed May 2010).

Reinberg, Steven. "Obesity While Young Boosts Pancreatic Cancer Risk." *U.S. News & World Report Health*, June 23, 2009. http://health.usnews.com/health-news/family-health/cancer/articles/2009/06/23/obesity-while-young-boosts-pancreatic-cancer-risk.html (accessed February 2010).

Reuters. "Animal Protein and Fat Raise Endometrial Cancer Risk." Reuters Health, March 21, 2007. http://www.reuters.com/article/idUSCOL16846020070321 (accessed April 2010).

Robbins, John. *Healthy at 100: How You Can — At Any Age — Dramatically Increase Your Life Span and Your Health Span.* New York: Random House, 2006.

Roth, Mark. "Cancer Expert Tells How Treatment Can Be Problem." *Pittsburgh Post-Gazette*, February 24, 2010.

Science*Daily*. "Chemical in Plastic Bottles Raises Some Concern." Science*Daily*, April 22, 2008. http://www.sciencedaily.com/releases/2008/04/080422114734.htm (accessed April 2010).

———. "Obesity Ups Cancer Risks, and Here's How." Science*Daily*, January 25, 2010. http://www.sciencedaily.com/releases/2010/01/100121135713.htm (accessed April 2010).

Singletary, Keith W., and Susan M. Gapstur. "Alcohol and Breast Cancer: Review of Epidemiologic and Experimental Evidence and Potential Mechanisms." *Journal of the American Medical Association* 286, no. 17 (November 2001). http://jama.ama-assn.org/cgi/content/abstract/286/17/2143 (accessed March 2010).

Sjödahl, K., C. Jia, L. Vatten, T. Nilsen, K. Hveem, and J. Lagergren. "Salt and Gastric Adenocarcinoma: A Population-based Cohort Study in Norway." *Cancer Epidemiology, Biomarkers and Prevention* 17, no. 8 (August 2008). http://www.ncbi.nlm.nih.gov/pubmed/18708389 (accessed April 2010).

Stein, Rob. "Daily Red Meat Raises Chances of Dying Early." *Washington Post Health*, March 24, 2009. http://www.washingtonpost.com/wp-dyn/content/article/2009/03/23/AR2009032301626.html (accessed February 2010).

United Press International. "WHO: Tanning Beds Can Cause Cancer." *UPI Health*, July 29, 2009. http://www.upi.com/Health_News/2009/07/29/WHO-Tanning-beds-can-cause-cancer/UPI-23981248842118/ (accessed April 2010).

University of California at Berkeley. "Wellness Guide to Dietary Supplements." UC Berkeley Wellness Letter, 2010. http://www.wellnessletter.com/html/ds/dsFishOil.php (accessed April 2010).

Ursin, G., E. Bjelke, I. Heuch, and S. E. Vollset. "Milk Consumption and Cancer Incidence: A Norwegian Prospective Study." *British Journal of Cancer* 61, no. 3 (March 1990). http://www.ncbi.nlm.nih.gov/pmc/articles/PMC1971283/ (accessed April 2010).

U.S. Food and Drug Administration. "Acrylamide Questions and Answers." FDA Web site, last updated May 13, 2009. http://www.fda.gov/Food/FoodSafety/FoodContaminantsAdulteration/ChemicalContaminants/Acrylamide/ucm053569.htm (accessed April 2010).

Vos Iz Neias. "Barcelona, Spain — Researchers: One-third of Breast Cancer May Be Avoidable." Vos Iz Neias, March 25, 2010. http://www.vosizneias.com/52090/2010/03/25/barcelona-spain-researchers-one-third-of-breast-cancer-may-be-avoidable (accessed April 2010).

Walsh, T. J., M. Schembri, P. J. Turek, J. M. Chan, P. R. Carroll, J. F. Smith, M. L. Eisenberg, S. K. Van Den Eeden, and M. S. Croughan. "Increased Risk of High-Grade Prostate Cancer among Infertile Men." *Cancer* 116, no. 9 (May 1, 2010). http://www.ncbi.nlm.nih.gov/pubmed/20309846 (accessed April 2010).

Wasserman, Harvey, and Norman Solomon. *Killing Our Own: The Disaster with America's Experience with Atomic Radiation.* New York: Delta/Dell, 1982. http://www.ratical.com/radiation/KillingOurOwn/KOO6.html (accessed April 2010).

Weil, Andrew. "Balancing Omega-3 and Omega-6?" Weil Q & A Library, February 2, 2007. http://www.drweil.com/drw/u/QAA400149/balancing-omega-3-and-omega-6.html (accessed April 2010).

————. "Is Eating Grapefruit a Breast Cancer Risk?" Weil Q & A Library, May 23, 2008. http://www.drweil.com/drw/u/QAA400404/Is-Eating-Grapefruit-a-Breast-Cancer-Risk.html (accessed April 2010).

Wikipedia, s.v. "Free-Radical Theory." http://en.wikipedia.org/wiki/Free-radical_theory (accessed April 2010).

Wolinsky, Howard. "Salty Diet Tied to Stomach Cancer in Korean Study." Reuters, March 24, 2010. http://www.reuters.com/article/idUSTRE62N4KX20100324 (accessed April 2010).

World Health Organization. "Global Cancer Rates Could Increase by 50% to 15 Million by 2020." April 3, 2003. http://www.who.int/mediacentre/news/releases/2003/pr27/en/ (accessed April 2010).

Youngman, L. D., and T. C. Campbell. "High Protein Intake Promotes the Growth of Preneoplastic Foci in Fischer #344 Rats: Evidence That Early Remodeled Foci Retain the Potential for Future Growth." *Journal of Nutrition* 121, no. 9 (September 1991): 1454-61.

————. "Inhibition of Aflatoxin B1-induced Gamma-glutamyltranspeptidase Positive (GGT+) Hepatic Preneoplastic Foci and Tumors by Low Protein Diets: Evidence That Altered GGT+ Foci Indicate Neoplastic Potential." *Carcinogenesis* 13, no. 9 (September 1992): 1607.

Zelman, Kathleen. "Organic Food — Is 'Natural' Worth the Extra Cost?" MedicineNet, August 7, 2007. http://www.medicinenet.com/script/main/art.asp?articlekey=52420 (accessed April 2010).

Chapter Notes

Introduction

1. T. Colin Campbell and Thomas M. Campbell II, *The China Study: Startling Implications for Diet, Weight Loss, and Long-term Health* (Dallas, TX: BenBella Books, 2006).

Chapter 1

1. National Cancer Institute, "SEER Stat Fact Sheets: All Sites," Surveillance Epidemiology and End Results (SEER). http://seer.cancer.gov/statfacts/html/all.html

2. Sharon Begley, "We Fought Cancer...and Cancer Won," *Newsweek* (September 6, 2008), http://www.newsweek.com/2008/09/05/we-fought-cancer-and-cancer-won.html.

3. Ahmedin Jemal and others, "Cancer Statistics 2008," *A Cancer Journal for Clinicians* 58 (February 20, 2008), http://caonline.amcancersoc.org/cgi/content/full/58/2/71

4. National Cancer Institute, "SEER Stat Fact Sheets: All Sites."

5. Clifton Leaf, "Why We're Losing the War on Cancer." Fortune (March 22, 2004), http://money.cnn.com/magazines/fortune/fortune_archive/2004/03/22/365076/index.htm.

6. Ibid.

7. National Cancer Institute, *SEER Fact Sheet*.

8. Leaf, "Why We're Losing the War on Cancer."

9. Ibid.

10. Ibid.

11. Ibid.

12. Ibid.

13. John McDougall, "The Fallacy of Early Detection," Keynote Address, McDougall Advanced Study Lecture Series, Santa Rosa, CA, February 20, 2010.

Chapter 2

1. Robert Krulwich, "Bacteria Outnumber Cells in Human Body," National Public Radio Website, July 1, 2006, http://www.npr.org/templates/story/story.php?storyId=5527426.

2. Alvis Brazma and others, "A Quick Introduction to Elements of Biology - Cells, Molecules, Genes, Functional Genomics,

Microarrays," European Bioinformatics Institute, October 2001, http://www.ebi.ac.uk/microarray/biology_intro.html

3. American Cancer Society, Oncogenes and Tumor Suppressor Genes," http://www.cancer.org/docroot/eto/content/eto_1_4x_oncogenes_and_tumor_suppressor_genes.asp.

4. Ibid.

5. Ibid.

6. Ibid.

7. Ibid.

8. Ibid.

9. Ibid.

10. National Institutes of Health, "Teacher's Guide: Understanding Cancer," http://science-education.nih.gov/supplements/nih1/Cancer/guide/understanding2.htm.

11. Ibid.

12. Ibid.

13. BioInfoBank Library, "Molecular Pathology of Cancer Cell," http://lib.bioinfo.pl/courses/view/158.

14. Peter Crosta, "What Is Cancer? What Causes Cancer?," *Medical News Today*, n.d., http://www.medicalnewstoday.com/info/cancer-oncology/whatiscancer.php.

15. Campbell and Campbell, *The China Study*, 48.

16. McDougall, "The Fallacy of Early Detection."

17. Ibid.

18. Campbell and Campbell, *The China Study*, 50.

Chapter 3

1. Healthcommunities.com, "Overview, Types of Bladder Cancer, Incidence," June 15, 1998, http://www.urologychannel.com/bladdercancer/index.shtml.

2. New Jersey Department of Health and Senior Services, "Cancer Risk Factors," http://www.statenj.us/health/cancer/cariskfactorsfsfinal02.htm.

3. Medline Plus Encyclopedia, "Schistosomiasis," http://www.nlm.nih.gov/medlineplus/ency/article/001321.htm.

4. Randy Dotinga, "Meat Lovers Face Greater Risk of Bladder

Cancer," Bloomberg Businessweek, April 20, 2010, http://www. businessweek.com/lifestyle/content/healthday/638268.html.

5. New Jersey Department of Health, "Cancer Risk Factors."

6. Cancer Project, "Ask the Expert: Eggs," http://www.cancerproject. org/ask/eggs.php.

7. J. C. Balbi and others, "Foods and Risk of Bladder Cancer: A Case-control Study in Uruguay," *European Journal of Cancer Prevention*, 10, no. 5 (October 2001), http://ncbi.nlm.nih.gov/pubmed/11711760.

8. Medline Plus Encyclopedia, "Brain Tumor – Primary – Adults," http://www.nlm.nih.gov/medlineplus/ency/article/007222.htm.

9. Ibid.

10. W. Lijinsky, "N-Nitroso compounds in the diet," *Mutation Research* 443, no. 1–2 (July 15, 1999), http://www.ncbi.nlm.nih.gov/ pubmed/10415436.

11. Michelle Conlin, "Cellphones Cause Brain Tumors, Says New Report by International EMF Collaborative," *Bloomberg Businessweek*, August 26, 2009, http://www.businessweek.com/ careers/managementiq/archives/2009/08/cellphones_caus.html.

12. Medline Plus Encyclopedia, Brain Tumor.

13. M. P. W. A. Houben and others, "Hypertension as a Risk Factor for Glioma? Evidence from a Population-based Study of Comorbidity in Glioma Patients," *Oxford Journal: Annals of Oncology* 15, no. 8 (2004), http://www.annonc.oxfordjournals.org/content/15/8/1256. abstract.

14. Russell Blaylock, *Natural Strategies for Cancer Patients,* (New York: Twin Streams/Kensington, 2003), 23.

15. American Cancer Society, "What Are the Key Statistics for Breast Cancer?" http://our.cancer.org/docroot/cri/content/cri_2_4_1x_ what_are_the_key_statistics_for_breast_cancer_5.asp.

16. Campbell and Campbell, *The China Study*, 161.

17. New Jersey Department of Health, "Cancer Risk Factors."

18. Ibid.

19. Campbell and Campbell, *The China Study*, 159.

20. Alona Pulde and Matthew Lederman, *Keep It Simple, Keep It Whole: Your Guide to Optimum Health* (Los Angeles, CA, USA: Exsalus Health & Wellness Center, 2009), 72.

21. Neal D. Barnard and Jennifer K. Reilly, *The Cancer Survivor's*

Guide: Foods That Help You Fight Back (Summertown, TN: Healthy Living Publications, 2008), 18.

22. Barnard and Reilly, *The Cancer Survivor's Guide*, 19.
23. Barnard and Reilly, *The Cancer Survivor's Guide*, 69.
24. American Cancer Society, "What Are the Risk Factors for Cervical Cancer?" http://our.cancer.org/docroot/cri/content/cri_2_4_2x_what_are_the_risk_factors_for_cervical_cancer_8.asp.
25. Ibid.
26. Blaylock, *Natural Strategies*, 10.
27. New Jersey Department of Health, "Cancer Risk Factors."
28. Campbell and Campbell, *The China Study*, 170.
29. Nancy J. Nelson, "Nurses' Health Study: Nurses Helping Science and Themselves," *Journal of the National Cancer Institute* 92. no. 8 (April 19, 2000), 597–599.
30. Campbell and Campbell, *The China Study*, 174.
31. Pulde and Lederman, *Keep It Simple*, 89.
32. Barnard and Reilly, *The Cancer Survivor's Guide*, 69.
33. Ibid., 25.
34. Ibid., 75.
35. Ibid.
36. Medline Plus Encyclopedia, "Endometrial Cancer," http://www.nlm.nih.gov/medlineplus/ency/article/000910.htm.
37. New Jersey Department of Health, "Cancer Risk Factors."
38. Ibid.
39. Reuters, "Animal Protein and Fat Raise Endometrial Cancer Risk," *Reuters Health,* March 21, 2007, http://www.reuters.com/article/idUSCOL16846020070321.
40. New Jersey Department of Health, "Cancer Risk Factors."
41. Neal D. Barnard, *"Foods That Fight Pain*: Revolutionary New Strategies for Maximum Pain Relief"* (New York: Three Rivers Press, 1998), 160.
42. New Jersey Department of Health, "Cancer Risk Factors."
43. American Cancer Society, "What Are the Risk Factors for Gallbladder Cancer?" http://our.cancer.org/docroot/cri/content/cri_2_4_2x_what_are_the_risk_factors_for_gall_bladder_cancer_68.asp.
44. New Jersey Department of Health, "Cancer Risk Factors."

45. American Cancer Society, What are the risk factors for laryngeal and hypopharyngeal cancer? http://our.cancer.org/docroot/cri/content/cri_2_4_2x_what_are_the_risk_factors_for_laryngeal_and_hypopharyngeal_cancer_23.asp.

46. M. A. Qadeer and others, Is GERD a Risk Factor for *Laryngeal Cancer? " Laryngoscope* 115, no. 3 (March 2005), http://www.ncbi.nlm.nih.gov/pubmed/15744163.

47. New Jersey Department of Health, "Cancer Risk Factors."

48. Leukemia & Lymphoma Society, "Facts and Statistics," July 1, 2009, http://www.leukemia-lymphoma.org/all_page?item_id=12486.

49. New Jersey Department of Health, "Cancer Risk Factors."

50. Life Extension, "Health Concerns: Leukemia." http://www.lef.org/protocols/cancer/leukemia_01.htm.

51. Ibid.

52. Wasserman, Harvey, and Norman Solomon. *Killing Our Own: The Disaster with America's Experience with Atomic Radiation.* New York: Delta/Dell, 1982. http://www.ratical.com/radiation/KillingOurOwn/KOO6.html.

53. Life Extension, *Health Concerns: Leukemia.*

54. Ibid.

55. Ibid.

56. Blaylock, *Natural Strategies*, 242.

57. Cancer Project, The, "Cancer Facts - Meat Consumption and Cancer Risk." http://www.cancerproject.org/diet_cancer/facts/meat.php.

58. Campbell and Campbell, *The China Study,* 104.

59. ScienceDaily, "Obesity Ups Cancer Risks, and Here's How," ScienceDaily, January 25, 2010, http://www.sciencedaily.com/releases/2010/01/100121135713.htm.

60. New Jersey Department of Health, "Cancer Risk Factors."

61. Jane E. Brody, "Huge Study Of Diet Indicts Fat And Meat," *New York Times Science*, May 8, 1990, http://www.nytimes.com/1990/05/08/science/huge_study_of_diet_indicts_fat_and_meat.html?pagewanted=1.

62. Ibid.

63. Centers for Disease Control and Prevention, "Lung Cancer Risk

Factors," http://www.cdc.gov/cancer/lung/basic_info/risk_factors. htm.

64. Ibid.

65. Ibid.

66. Ibid.

67. MedicineNet.com, "Hodgkin's Disease Adult," http://www. medicinenet.com/hodgkins_disease/article.htm.

68. American Cancer Society, *What Causes Hodgkin Disease?*" http:// our.cancer.org/docroot/CRI/content/CRI_2_2_2X_What_causes_ Hodgkins_disease_Can_it_be_prevented_20.asp.

69. Karen Barrow, The Link between Rheumatoid Arthritis and Lymphoma," ScienceDaily, November 17, 2009, http://sciencedaily. healthology.com/arthritis/article3960.htm.

70. Ibid.

71. G. Ursin and others, Milk Consumption and Cancer Incidence: A Norwegian Prospective Study ," *British Journal of Cancer* 61, no. 3 (March 1990), http://www.ncbi.nlm.nih.gov/pmc/articles/ PMC1971283/.

72. MedicineNet, Non-Hodgkin's Lymphoma (cont.), http://www. medicinenet.com/non-hodgkins_lymphomas/page2.htm.

73. Ibid.

74. John McDougall, "Low Vitamin D: One Sign of Sunlight Deficiency," *McDougall Newsletter*, September 2007, http:// drmcdougall.com/misc/2007nl/sep/070900.pdf.

75. New Jersey Department of Health.

76. United Press International, "WHO: Tanning Beds Can Cause Cancer," *UPI Health*, July 29, 2009, http://www.upi.com/Health_ News/2009/07/29/WHO-Tanning-beds-can-cause-cancer/UPI- 23981248842118/.

77. Melanoma Center, "Risk Factors: Suppressed Immune System," http://www.melanomacenter.org/risk/sis.html.

78. John McDougall, "Sunny Days, Keeping Those Clouds Away...." *McDougall Newsletter*, May 2005, http://wwwdrmcdougall.com/misc/ pdf/pdf050500nl.pdf.

79. New Jersey Department of Health, "Cancer Risk Factors."

80. National Health Service, "Mouth Cancer: Are You at Risk?" http:// www.nhs.uk/Livewell/cancer/Pages/Mouthcancer.aspx.

81. Mouth Cancer Foundation, Reduce Your Chances of Getting These Cancers By:" http://www.rdoc.org.uk/.

82. Claudia Frias, Oral sex linked to increased cancer rates in young people," *TerraUSA*, April 16, 2010, http://en.terra.com/dating-relationships/news/oral_sex_linked_to_increased_cancer_rates_in_young_people/hof9149.

83. New Jersey Department of Health, "Cancer Risk Factors."

84. National Research Council, Committee on Diet and Health, *Diet and Health: Implications for Reducing Chronic Disease Risk.* (Washington, DC: National Academies Press, 1989), http://books.nap.edu/openbook.php?record_id=1222&page=599.

85. Barnard, *Foods That Fight Pain*, 157.

86. Ibid., 158.

87. Ibid.

88. Ibid.

89. Ibid.

90. Barnard and Reilly, *The Cancer Survivor's Guide,* 19.

91. Lawrence H. Kushi and others, Prospective Study of Diet and Ovarian Cancer," *American Journal of Epidemiology* 149, no. 1 (January 1, 1999), http://www.ncbi.nlm.nih.gov/pubmed/9883790.

92. Cancer Research UK. "Pancreatic Cancer Risks and Causes." http://www.cancerhelp.org.uk/type/pancreatic-cancer/about/pancreatic-cancer-risks-and-causes.

93. Health Communities, Pancreatic Cancer Risk Factors," August 15, 1999, http://www.oncologychannel.com/pancreaticcancer/risk-factors.shtml.

94. Agence France-Presse (AFP), "Sugary Soft Drinks Linked to Pancreatic Cancer," *Bangkok Post*, February 9, 2010, http://www.bangkokpost.com/news/health/167914/sugary-soft-drinks-linked-to-pancreatic-cancer-study.

95. Ibid.

96. Steven Reinberg, "Obesity While Young Boosts Pancreatic Cancer Risk," *U.S. News & World Report Health*, June 23, 2009, http://health.usnews.com/health-news/family-health/cancer/articles/2009/06/23/obesity-while-young-boosts-pancreatic-cancer-risk.html.

97. Campbell and Campbell, *The China Study*, 177.

98. Ibid, 178.

99. Ibid.

100. Ibid., 367.

101. Ibid., 179.

102. T. J. Walsh and others, "Increased risk of high-grade prostate cancer among infertile men," *Cancer* 116, no. 9 (May 1, 2010), http://www.ncbi.nlm.nih.gov/pubmed/20309846.

103. New Jersey Department of Health, "Cancer Risk Factors."

104. K. Sjödahl, Salt and gastric adenocarcinoma: a population-based cohort study in Norway," *Cancer Epidemiology, Biomarkers and Prevention* 17, no. 8 (August 2008), http://www.ncbi.nlm.nih.gov/pubmed/18708389.

105. McDougall, "Salt, The Scapegoat for the Western Diet."

106. National Cancer Institute, "Heterocyclic Amines in Cooked Meats," http://www.cancer.gov/cancertopics/factsheet/Risk/heterocyclic-amines.

107. Lawrence H. Kushi, ScD, and others, "American Cancer Society Guidelines on Nutrition and Physical Activity for Cancer Prevention." ," *CA: A Cancer Journal for Clinicians* 56 (September–October 2006), http://caonline.amcancersoc.org/cgi/content/full/56/5/254.

108. New Jersey Department of Health, "Cancer Risk Factors."

109. John McDougall, "Soy—Food, WonderDrug or Poison?" *McDougall Newsletter*, April 2005. http://www.drmcdougall.com/misc/2005nl/april/050400pusoy.htm.

110. Medical News Today. "Multiple Dental X-Rays Raise Risk of Thyroid Cancer." http://www.medicalnewstoday.com/articles/191025.php.

Chapter 4

1. Dana-Farber Cancer Institute, Cancer Prevention Quick Facts" (sidebar on "February: National Cancer Prevention Month" page), http://www.dana-farber.org/can/monthly-cancer-awareness/national-cancer-prevention-month/.

2. Barnard, *Foods That Fight Pain,* 150.

3. Cancer Research UK, "What Causes Cancer?" http://www.cancerhelp.org.uk/about-cancer/causes-symptoms/causes/what-causes-cancer.

4. New Jersey Department of Health, "Cancer Risk Factors."

5. John Mackey, "Whole Foods Markets' Efforts to Change the World through Better Nutrition," Presentation, McDougall Advanced Study Lecture Series, Santa Rosa, CA, February 19, 2010.

6. Blaylock, *Natural Strategies*, 46.

7. Ibid., 47.

8. Ibid., 46.

9. Keith Singletary, and Susan M. Gapstur, "Alcohol and Breast Cancer: Review of Epidemiologic and Experimental Evidence and Potential Mechanisms," *Journal of the American Medical Association*, 286, no. 17 (November 2001), http://jama.ama-assn.org/cgi/content/abstract/286/17/2143.

10. Jack Challem, "Beating Breast Cancer: If Genes Don't Matter, What Does?" *Nutrition Reporter*, 2000, http://www.thenutritionreporter.com/beating_breast_cancer.html.

11. Medicineworld.org, "What Causes Cancer?" http://medicineworld.org/cancer/page14.html.

12. National Cancer Institute, "Alcohol and Breast Cancer Risk: New Findings," http://www.cancer.gov/cancertopics/causes/breast/alcoholuse0408.

13. American Cancer Society, "Common Questions about Diet and Cancer," http://our.cancer.org/docroot/PED/content/PED_3_2X_Common_Questions_About_Diet_and_Cancer.asp.

14. National Cancer Institute, "Acrylamide in Food and Cancer Risk," http://www.cancer.gov/cancertopics/factsheet/risk/acrylamide-in-food.

15. U.S. Food and Drug Administration, "Acrylamide Questions and Answers," FDA Web site, last updated May 13, 2009, http://www.fda.gov/Food/FoodSafety/FoodContaminantsAdulteration/ChemicalContaminants/Acrylamide/ucm053569.htm.

16. Ibid.

17. Ibid.

18. John McDougall, "Acrylamide Poisoning: Cancer from Overcooked Carbohydrates?" *McDougall Newsletter*, June 2005, http://www.drmcdougall.com/misc/2005nl/june/050600acrylamide.htm.

19. Blaylock, *Natural Strategies*, 138.

20. National Cancer Institute, "HIV Infection and Cancer Risk," http://

www.cancer.gov/cancertopics/factsheet/risk/hiv-infection.

21. Campbell and Campbell, *The China Study,* 79.

22. American Heart Association, *What Your Cholesterol Levels Mean.*

23. Campbell and Campbell, *The China Study,* 78.

24. Ibid.

25. Ibid., 80.

26. Barnard and Reilly, *The Cancer Survivor's Guide*, 40.

27. Pulde and Lederman, *Keep It Simple,* 71.

28. Barnard and Reilly, *The Cancer Survivor's Guide*, 40.

29. June M. Chan and others, "Dairy Products, Calcium, and Prostate Cancer Risk in the Physicians' Health Study," *American Journal of Clinical Nutrition* 74, no. 4 (October 2001), http://www.ajcn.org/cgi/content/full/74/4/549.

30. Barnard and Reilly, *The Cancer Survivor's Guide*, 18.

31. Ibid., viii.

32. Campbell and Campbell, *The China Study,* 6.

33. Barnard and Reilly, *The Cancer Survivor's Guide*, viii.

34. Campbell and Campbell, *The China Study,* 65.

35. Barnard and Reilly, *The Cancer Survivor's Guide*, 48.

36. Campbell and Campbell, *The China Study,* 87.

37. Ibid., 89.

38. Ibid.

39. Blaylock, *Natural Strategies,* 239.

40. National Cancer Institute, "Fluoridated Water: Questions and Answers," http://www.cancer.gov/cancertopics/factsheet/Risk/fluoridated-water.

41. National Cancer Institute, "Artificial Sweeteners and Cancer," http://www.cancer.gov/cancertopics/factsheet/Risk/artificial-sweeteners.

42. Christine H. Farlow, "Do You Eat Food With Any Of These 9 Cancer-Causing Chemicals?" *Healthy Eating Advisor*, 2004, http://www.healthyeatingadvisor.com/9cancer-causingchemicals.html.

43. Tricia Ellis-Christensen, What is Carrageenan? " Wisegeek, n.d., http://www.wisegeek.com/what-is-carrageenan.htm.

44. Barnard and Reilly, *The Cancer Survivor's Guide,* viii.

45. Ibid.

46. Campbell and Campbell, *The China Study,* 102.

47. Blaylock, *Natural Strategies,* 49.

48. Ibid.

49. Wikipedia , s.v., *Free Radical Theory,*" http://en.wikipedia.org/wiki/Free-radical_theory.

50. Blaylock, *Natural Strategies,* 42.

51. Ibid.

52. HealthCheck Systems, "Understanding Free Radicals and Antioxidants," http://www.healthchecksystems.com/antioxid.htm.

53. Campbell and Campbell, *The China Study,* 219.

54. Blaylock, *Natural Strategies,* 45.

55. Barnard and Reilly, *The Cancer Survivor's Guide,* ix.

56. Andrew Weil, Is Eating Grapefruit a Breast Cancer Risk? " Weil Q & A Library, May 23, 2008, http://www.drweil.com/drw/u/QAA400404/Is-Eating-Grapefruit-a-Breast-Cancer-Risk.html.

57. Ibid.

58. Ibid.

59. Campbell and Campbell, *The China Study,* 87.

60. DNA Direct, "Who Is At Risk for Ovarian Cancer?" http://www.dnadirect.com/web/article/testing-for-genetic-disorders/breast-and-ovarian-cancer-risk/93/who-is-at-risk-for-ovarian-cancer.

61. National Cancer Institute, "BRCA1 and BRCA2: Cancer Risk and Genetic Testing," http://www.cancer.gov/cancertopics/factsheet/Risk/BRCA.

62. Campbell and Campbell, *The China Study,* 161.

63. Ibid., 162.

64. Ibid., 159.

65. Ibid., 87.

66. Challem, "Beating Breast Cancer."

67. Ibid.

68. Campbell and Campbell, *The China Study,* 87.

69. Ibid.

70. Ibid., 88.

71. Ibid., 179.

72. McDougall, "Dr. McDougall Disputes Major Medical Treatments," DVD, 2007, John McDougall.

73. Campbell and Campbell, *The China Study,* 179.

74. McDougall, "Dr. McDougall Disputes Major Medical Treatments," DVD, 2007, John McDougall.

75. Blaylock, *Natural Strategies,* 197.

76. Ibid., 200.

77. Ibid., 195.

78. Ibid., 197.

79. Ibid., 198.

80. Ibid.

81. Ibid.

82. Barnard and Reilly, *The Cancer Survivor's Guide,* ix.

83. National Cancer Institute, Understanding Cancer Series: Cancer," http://www.cancer.gov/cancertopics/understandingcancer/cancer/allpages, Slide 60, Industrial Pollution.

84. National Cancer Institute, "Dioxins," Cancer Trends Progress Report: Dioxins. 2009–2010 Update, http://progressreport.cancer.gov/doc_detail.asp?pid=1&did=2009&chid=91&coid=914&mid=.

85. Lisa Fayed, "The Causes and Risk Factors of Cancer," About.com: Cancer, August 2006, http://cancer.about.com/od/causes/a/causesrisks.htm.

86. Ibid.

87. National Cancer Institute, "Pesticides," Cancer Trends Progress Report. 2009–2010 Update, http://progressreport.cancer.gov/doc_detail.asp?pid=1&did=2009&chid=91&coid=913&mid=.

88. Pulde and Lederman, Keep It Simple, 72.

89. Consumers Union, "Concern Over Canned Foods." Consumer Reports, December 2009, http://www.consumerreports.org/cro/magazine-archive/december-2009/food/bpa/overview/bisphenol-a-ov.htm.

90. Science*Daily*, "Chemical In Plastic Bottles Raises Some Concern," Science*Daily*, April 22, 2008, http://www.sciencedaily.com/releases/2008/04/080422114734.htm.

91. Ibid.

92. Cancer Research UK, "What Causes Cancer?"

93. Fayed, "The Causes and Risk Factors of Cancer."

94. Newcomb-Fernandez, "Cancer in the HIV-Infected Population."

95. Cancer Research UK, "What Causes Cancer?"

96. Ibid.

97. National Cancer Institute, *"H. pylori and Cancer."*

98. American Cancer Society, "Chronic Inflammation Linked to Cancer," http://our.cancer.org/docroot/NWS/content/NWS_1_1x_ Chronic_Inflammation_Linked_to_Cancer.asp.

99. Ibid.

100. Blaylock, *Natural Strategies,* 50.

101. Ibid, 49.

102. John McDougall, "A Starch-based Diet Supports Spontaneous Healing: Atherosclerosis, Arthritis, and Sometimes Cancer," *McDougall Newsletter*, May 2009, http://www.drmcdougall.com/ misc/2009nl/may/090500.pdf.

103. Ibid.

104. George J. Brewer, "Risks of Copper and Iron Toxicity during Aging in Humans," *Chemical Research in Toxicology* 23, no. 2 (December 7, 2009), http://pubs.acs.org/doi/abs/10.1021/tx900338d.

105. Cancer Project, The, "Diet and Cancer Research—Iron: the Double-Edged Sword, http://www.cancerproject.org/diet_cancer/ nutrition/iron.php.

106. Ibid.

107. Ibid.

108. John McDougall, "Favorite Five Articles from Recent Medical Journals," *McDougall Newsletter,* March 2010, http://www. drmcdougall.com/misc/2010nl/mar/fav5.htm.

109. Campbell and Campbell, *The China Study,* 94.

110. Ibid, 180.

111. Ibid.

112. Barnard and Reilly, *The Cancer Survivor's Guide,* 26.

113. Ibid.

114. Ibid.

115. Rob Stein, "Daily Red Meat Raises Chances of Dying Early," Washington Post Health, March 24, 2009, http:// www.washingtonpost.com/wp-dyn/content/article/2009/03/23/ AR2009032301626.html.

116. Ibid.

117. Blaylock, Natural Strategies, 20.

118. Ibid, 49.

119. Ibid.

120. Mackey, "Whole Foods Markets' Efforts to Change the World through Better Nutrition."

121. Challem, "Beating Breast Cancer."

122. National Cancer Institute, "Obesity and Cancer: Questions and Answers," http://www.cancer.gov/cancertopics/factsheet/Risk/obesity.

123. Ibid.

124. Ibid.

125. Ibid.

126. Blaylock, *Natural Strategies,* 135.

127. Ibid.

128. John McDougall, "New Trans-Fat Labels : Too Little, Too Late," Dr. McDougall's Health and Medical Center Web site, http://www.drmcdougall.com/res_trans_fat_labels.html.

129. McDougall, "Sunny Days, Keeping Those Clouds Away..."

130. New York Times Health Guide, "Physical Activity: Exercise's Effects on Other Conditions," *New York Times Health*, March 1, 2009, http://health.nytimes.com/health/guides/specialtopic/physical-activity/exercise's-effects-on-other-conditions.html.

131. Ibid.

132. Ibid.

133. Ibid.

134. United Press International, "WHO: Tanning beds can cause cancer."

135. American Cancer Society, "Can Cancer be Prevented?"

136. American Cancer Society, "Tobacco-Related Cancers Fact Sheet."

137. Challem, "Beating Breast Cancer."

138. American Cancer Society, "Tobacco-Related Cancers Fact Sheet."

139. American Cancer Society, "Can Cancer be Prevented?"

140. American Cancer Society, "Tobacco-Related Cancers Fact Sheet."

141. Blaylock, *Natural Strategies,* 19.

142. Challem, "Beating Breast Cancer."

143. Blaylock, *Natural Strategies,* 202.

144. Ibid, 35.

145. "Anesthesia May Affect Metastasis Risk after Cancer Surgery," *Journal of Anaesthesiology Clinical Pharmacology.* online report, http://www.joacp.org/index.php?option=com_content&view=article&id=60&catid=1.

146. McDougall, "New Trans-Fat Labels for 2006."

147. Ibid.

Chapter 5

1. Barnard, *Foods That Fight Pain*, 147.

2. Ibid.

3. Ibid.

4. Barnard, Foods That Fight Pain, 148.

5. Ibid.

6. Ibid.

7. Barnard, Foods That Fight Pain, 149.

8. Pritikin Longevity Center and Spa, Nathan Pritikin : Founder, The Pritikin Program," http://www.pritikin.com/index.php?option=com_content&view=article&id=61&Itemid=89.

9. Ibid.

10. Ibid.

11. Ibid.

12. Ibid.

13. Campbell and Campbell, *The China Study,* 5.

14. Ibid.

15. Ibid, 56.

16. Ibid, 50.

17. Gio B. Gori, "Diet and Nutrition in Cancer Causation," *Nutrition and Cancer: An International Journal* 1, no. 1 (Fall 1978), 5.

18. Ivan Oransky, "Sir Richard Doll," *The Lancet* 366, no. 9434 (August 6, 2005), http://www.thelancet.com/journals/lancet/article/PIIS0140-6736(05)67047-X/fulltext.

19. G. E. Dunaif and T. C. Campbell, "Relative Contribution of Dietary Protein Level and Aflatoxin B_1 Dose in Generation of Presumptive Preneoplastic Foci in Rat Liver," *Journal of the National Cancer Institute* 78, no. 2 (February 1987), 365, http://www.ncbi.nlm.nih.gov/

---

pubmed/3100852.

20. L. D. Youngman and T. C. Campbell. "High Protein Intake Promotes the Growth of Preneoplastic Foci in Fischer #344 Rats," : Evidence That Early Remodeled Foci Retain the Potential for Future Growth," *Journal of Nutrition* 121, no. 9 (September 1991), 1454, http://www.ncbi.nlm.nih.gov/pubmed/1679128.

21. L. D. Youngman and T. C. Campbell. "Inhibition of Aflatoxin B_1-induced Gamma-glutamyltranspeptidase Positive (GGT+) Hepatic Preneoplastic Foci and Tumors by Low Protein Diets,": Evidence That Altered GGT+ Foci Indicate Neoplastic Potential," *Carcinogenesis* 13, no. 9 (September 1992), 1607, http://carcin. oxfordjournals.org/cgi/content/abstract/13/9/1607.

22. Campbell and Campbell, *The China Study,* 61.

23. John Robbins, *Healthy at 100*: *How You Can — At Any Age — Dramatically Increase Your Life Span and Your Health Span* (New York: Random House, 2006) 125.

24. Campbell and Campbell, *The China Study,* 70.

25. Robbins, *Healthy at 100*, 126.

26. Campbell and Campbell, *The China Study,* 73.

27. Ibid.

28. Robbins, *Healthy at 100*, 124.

29. Ibid.

30. Ibid.

31. Robbins, *Healthy at 100*, 126.

32. Campbell and Campbell, *The China Study,* 73.

Chapter 6

1. McDougall, "The Fallacy of Early Detection."

2. Ibid.

3. Ibid.

4. Vos Iz Neias, "Barcelona, Spain—Researchers: One-third of Breast Cancer May be Avoidable," *Vos Iz Neias*, March 25, 2010, http://www.vosizneias.com/52090/2010/03/25/barcelona-spain-researchers-one-third-of-breast-cancer-may-be-avoidable.

5. American Cancer Society, "Nine Risk Factors Account for One-Third of World's Cancer Deaths," http://www.cancer.org/docroot/NWS/content/NWS_2_1x_Nine_Risk_Factors_Account_for_One-

Third_of_Worlds_Cancer_Deaths.asp.

6. World Health Organization, "Global Cancer Rates Could Increase by 50% to 15 Million by 2020," April 3, 2003, http://www.who.int/mediacentre/news/releases/2003/pr27/en/.

7. Blaylock, *Natural Strategies,* xvii.

8. Campbell and Campbell, *The China Study,* 97.

9. Ibid. 98.

10. Ibid. 99.

11. CitySpur, "How to Prevent Cancer—A Detailed Study," Long Beach 10 Web site, from an article posted on Meditrendz (http://www.meditrendz.com/archives/2009/how-to-prevent-cancer-a-detailed-study/), March 11, 2009, http://longbeach10.cityspur.com/2009/11/23/how-to-prevent-cancer-a-detailed-study/.

12. Ibid.

13. Ann Kulze, "Dr. Ann's 10-Steps to Prevent Breast Cancer," About.com Women's Health, last updated October 30, 2009, http://womenshealth.about.com/od/cancerprevention/a/10stepsprevbcan.htm.

14. Ibid.

15. CitySpur, "How to Prevent Cancer."

16. Ibid.

17. Kulze, "Dr. Ann's 10-Steps."

18. CitySpur, "How to Prevent Cancer."

19. Ibid.

20. Ibid.

21. Ibid.

22. Ibid.

23. Ibid.

24. Ibid.

25. Ibid.

26. Ibid.

27. Kulze, "Dr. Ann's 10-Steps."

28. Ibid.

29. CitySpur, "How to Prevent Cancer."

30. ReadersDigest.com, "Top 10 Antioxidant-Rich Fruits and Veggies," http://www.rd.com/living-healthy/top-10-antioxidant-rich-fruits-and-

veggies/article16245.html

31. Ibid.

32. Ibid.

33. Cancer Prevention Coalition, "International Scientific Committee Warns of Serious Risks of Breast and Prostate Cancer from Monsanto's Hormonal Milk," http://www.preventcancer.com/press/releases/march21_99.htm.

34. NutritionMD, "Making Sense of Foods: Understanding the Problems with Dairy Products," http://www.nutritionmd.org/nutrition_tips/nutrition_tips_understand_foods/dairy.html.

35. Daily Mail staff reporter, "Eating Tofu Can Slash Ovarian Cancer Risk," *Mail Online,* January 12, 2007, http://www.dailymail.co.uk/news/article-428478/Eating-tofu-slash-ovarian-cancer-risk.html.

36. Pulde and Lederman, *Keep It Simple,* 80.

37. Campbell and Campbell, *The China Study,* 170.

38. Kushi and others, "American Cancer Society Guidelines on Nutrition."

39. Desiree Jones, "Whole Grains Reduce Heart Disease 30 Percent, Diabetes in Women," Gibson's Healthful Living Blog, August 19, 2009. http://www.gibsonshealth.com/blog/?p=81.

40. Kushi and others, "American Cancer Society Guidelines on Nutrition."

41. Kulze, "Dr. Ann's 10-Steps."

42. Barnard and Reilly, *The Cancer Survivor's Guide,* 5.

43. Barnard and Reilly, *The Cancer Survivor's Guide,* 43.

44. Blaylock, *Natural Strategies,* 135.

45. Ban Trans Fat, "About Trans Fat," http://www.bantransfats.com/abouttransfat.html.

46. Howard Wolinsky, "Salty Diet Tied to Stomach Cancer in Korean Study," Reuters, March 24, 2010, http://www.reuters.com/article/idUSTRE62N4KX20100324.

47. Agence France-Presse, "Green Tea, Mushrooms Combat Cancer," *Bangkok Post,* March 18, 2009, http://www.bangkokpost.com/breakingnews/137800/green-tea-mushrooms-combat-cancer.

48. Agence France-Presse, "Red wine and dark chocolate cancer killers : Researcher," *Physorg,* February 11, 2010, http://www.physorg.com/news185087626.html.

49. Agence France-Presse, "Researchers Back Cancer-Fighting Properties of Papaya," *Vancouver Sun,* March 9, 2010, http://www. vancouversun.com/story_print.html?id=2662932&sponsor.

50. CitySpur, "How to Prevent Cancer."

51. Ibid.

52. Ibid.

53. Kulze, "Dr. Ann's 10-Steps."

54. CitySpur, "How to Prevent Cancer."

55. Ibid.

56. Loren Pickart, "The Chemical Sunscreen Health Disaster," http:// www.skinbiology.com/toxicsunscreens.html.

57. CitySpur, "How to Prevent Cancer."

58. Ibid.

59. CitySpur, "How to Prevent Cancer."

60. Ibid.

61. John McDougall, "Vitamin D Pills Are of Little or No Benefit and Some Harm So What to Do Now?" *McDougall Newsletter*, March 2010, http://www.drmcdougall.com/misc/2010nl/mar/vitd.htm.

62. CitySpur, "How to Prevent Cancer."

63. Kulze, "Dr. Ann's 10-Steps."

64. Ibid.

65. Mayo Clinic staff, "Cancer Prevention: Seven Steps to Reduce Your Risk."

66. Ibid.

67. CitySpur, "How to Prevent Cancer."

68. Mayo Clinic staff, "Cancer Prevention."

69. McDougall, "The Fallacy of Early Detection."

70. L. Lloyd Morgan, "Cellphones and Brain Tumors: 15 reasons for concern."

71. Matt Hamblen, "Cell Phone, Cancer Link Claimed," PC World, August 29, 2009, http://www.pcworld.com/article/171012/cell_phone_cancer_link_claimed.html.

72. Christopher Babayode, Wave Your Health Good-bye with Sky High WiFi," WEEP News, August 28, 2009, http://weepnews.blogspot. com/2009/08/thyroid-cancer-increase-puzzles-experts.html.

Chapter 7

1. Neal D. Barnard, "Breaking the Food Seduction," Presentation, McDougall Advanced Lecture Series, Santa Rosa, CA, February 19, 2010.

2. McDougall, "Dr. McDougall Disputes Major Medical Treatments."

3. Barnard and Reilly, *The Cancer Survivor's Guide,* 25.

4. Good Housekeeping staff, "About the Anti-Aging Diet," *Good Housekeeping Diet and Health*, 2010, http://www.goodhousekeeping. com/health/diet/about-anti-aging-diet.

5. McDougall, "Dr. McDougall Disputes Major Medical Treatments."

6. Ibid.

7. Ibid.

8. Barnard and Reilly, *The Cancer Survivor's Guide,* 4.

9. Ibid.

10. McDougall, "Dr. McDougall Disputes Major Medical Treatments."

11. John McDougall, "Dr. McDougall's Common Sense Nutrition," DVD, 2008, John McDougall.

12. McDougall, "Salt: The Scapegoat for the Western Diet."

13. Ibid.

14. Barnard and Reilly, *The Cancer Survivor's Guide,* 76.

15. Douglas Gansler, "A Deadly Ingredient in a Chicken Dinner," *Washington Post*, June 26, 2009, http://www.washingtonpost.com/wp-dyn/content/article/2009/06/25/AR2009062503381.html.

16. Kathy Freston, *Quantum Wellness: A Practical and Spiritual Guide to Health and Happiness*, (New York: Weinstein, 2008) 112.

17. Blaylock, *Natural Strategies,* 153.

18. Ibid. 27.

19. Ibid. 238.

20. Ibid. 27.

21. Barnard and Reilly, *The Cancer Survivor's Guide,* 69.

22. Ibid. 11.

23. Ibid. 10.

24. Ibid.

25. Ibid. 1.

26. Ibid. 72.

27. Maria Miller, "Omega-3 Fats and Intelligence," *Home School Math,* n.d., http://www.homeschoolmath.net/teaching/fats-intelligence.php.

28. Ibid.

29. Andrew Weil, *"Balancing Omega-3 and Omega-6?"* Weil Q & A Library, February 2, 2007, http://www.drweil.com/drw/u/ QAA400149/balancing-omega-3-and-omega-6.html.

30. Ibid.

31. Ibid.

32. Barnard and Reilly, *The Cancer Survivor's Guide,* 71.

33. John McDougall, "Vegan Diet Damages Baby's Brain - Sensationalism! People Love to Hear Good News about their Bad Habits!" *McDougall Newsletter,* February 2003, http://www. nealhendrickson.com/McDougall/030200puVeganDietDamages. htm.

34. Ibid.

35. Barnard and Reilly, *The Cancer Survivor's Guide,* 71.

36. Ibid.

37. Ibid. 72.

38. Ibid.

39. Ibid. viii.

40. Barnard, *Foods That Fight Pain*, 146.

41. Ibid. 153.

42. McDougall, "The Fallacy of Early Detection."

43. Ibid.

44. Ibid.

45. Blaylock, *Natural Strategies,* 9.

46. McDougall, "The Fallacy of Early Detection."

47. Campbell and Campbell, *The China Study,* 61.

48. Vos Iz Neias, "Barcelona, Spain."

49. Ibid.

50. Ibid.

51. Barnard and Reilly, *The Cancer Survivor's Guide,* 2.

52. Ibid.

53. Vos Iz Neias, "Barcelona, Spain."

54. Barnard and Reilly, *The Cancer Survivor's Guide,* vii.

55. Ibid.

56. Ibid. 2.

57. McDougall, "The Fallacy of Early Detection."

58. Ibid.

59. Ibid.

60. Maria Cheng, "Losing breast not always best for cancer patients," *Chicago Defender Online*, March 31, 2010, http://www.chicagodefender.com/article-7488-losing-breast-not-al.html.

61. Mark Roth, "Cancer Expert Tells How Treatment Can Be Problem," *Pittsburgh Post-Gazette*, February 24, 2010.

62. Barnard and Reilly, *The Cancer Survivor's Guide*, 2.

63. Barnard, *Foods That Fight Pain*, 150.

64. Campbell and Campbell, *The China Study*, 66.

65. T. Colin Campbell, "Hidden hazards of animal protein," McDougall Advanced Lecture Series, DVD, Produced by John and Mary McDougall, 2008.

66. Blaylock, *Natural Strategies*, 7.

67. Ibid. 74.

68. Ibid.

Chapter 8

1. McDougall, "Dr. McDougall's Common Sense Nutrition."

2. Ibid.

3. Ibid.

4. Reed Mangels, Protein in the Vegan Diet," The Vegetarian Resource Group (originally published in *Simply Vegan: Quick Vegetarian Meals* by Debra Wasserman and Reed Mangels), http://www.vrg.org/nutrition/protein.htm.

5. Nutritional Supplements, "Essential Amino Acids," http://www.glisonline.com/essential-amino-acids.html.

6. Mike Mahler, "Making the Vegan Diet Work," Mahler's Aggressive Strength Nutrition Articles, n.d., http://www.mikemahler.com/articles/vegan_diet.html.

7. Anne Collins, "Protein and Diet Information," http://www.annecollins.com/protein-diet.htm.

8. Campbell and Campbell, *The China Study*, 58.

9. Ibid. 37.

10. Mike Mahler, "Getting Big and Strong on a Vegan Diet," Bodybuilding, n.d., http://www.bodybuilding.com/fun/mahler53.htm.

11. Robert Cohen, "Who Gets Bone Disease?" http://www.sunfood.net/milk-bones.html.

12. Ibid.

13. McLean, *Milk – Calcium – Protein: Do they protect from osteoporosis?*

14. Ibid.

15. Campbell and Campbell, *The China Study*, 205.

16. Ibid., 211.

17. Cohen, *"Who Gets Bone Disease?"*

18. Ibid.

19. Rob McLean, "Milk – Calcium – Protein: Do They Protect from Osteoporosis?" Cyberparent.com, http://www.cyberparent.com/nutrition/osteoporosiscausemilk.htm.

20. Campbell and Campbell, *The China Study*, 3.

21. Ibid., 178.

22. Mark Bittman, "Eating Food That's Better for You, Organic or Not," *New York Times Week in Review*, March 21, 2009, http://www.nytimes.com/2009/03/22/weekinreview/22bittman.html.

23. Ibid.

24. Kathleen Zelman, *"Organic Food: Is 'Natural' Worth the Extra Cost?"* MedicineNet, August 7, 2007, http://www.medicinenet.com/script/main/art.asp?articlekey=52420.

25. Ibid.

26. Campbell and Campbell, *The China Study*, 235.

27. Bittman, "Eating Food That's Better for You, Organic or Not."

28. Zelman, "Organic Food: Is 'Natural' Worth the Extra Cost?"

29. McDougall, "My Favorite Five Articles."

30. Ibid.

31. McDougall, "Dr. McDougall's Common Sense Nutrition."

32. Ibid.

33. Ibid.

34. Bonnie Liebman, "Slow Burn: How Inflammation Can Trigger a Heart Attack," The Free Library (originally published in Nutrition Action Newsletter, January 1, 2009), http://www.thefreelibrary.com/

Slow+burn:+how+inflamation+can+trigger+a+heart+attack. -a0192898839.

35. National Library of Medicine, Medline Plus Medical Encyclopedia, C-reactive protein: http://www.nlm.nih.gov/medlineplus/ency/ article/003356.htm

36. Ibid.

37. McDougall, "Dr. McDougall's Common Sense Nutrition."

38. Ibid.

39. Marian Burros, "High Mercury Levels Are Found in Tuna Sushi," *New York Times Dining & Wine*, January 23, 2008, http://www. nytimes.com/2008/01/23/dining/23sushi.html.

40. University of California at Berkeley, "Wellness Guide to Dietary Supplements," UC Berkeley Wellness Letter, 2010, http://www. wellnessletter.com/html/ds/dsFishOil.php.

41. Barnard and Reilly, *The Cancer Survivor's Guide,* 38.

42. Melanoma Center, "Risk Factors."

43. Barnard and Reilly, *The Cancer Survivor's Guide,* 40.

44. John McDougall, "When Friends Ask: Why Do You Avoid Adding Vegetable Oils?" *McDougall Newsletter*, August 2007, http://www. drmcdougall.com/misc/2007nl/aug/oils.htm.

45. McDougall, "Dr. McDougall's Common Sense Nutrition."

46. McDougall, "When Friends Ask."

47. Campbell and Campbell, 228.

48. Ibid.

49. Kolata, "Vitamins: More May Be Too Many." *New York Times Science*, April 29, 2003, http://www.nytimes.com/2003/04/29/science/ vitamins-more-may-be-too-many.html?pagewanted=1.

50. Ibid.

51. Ibid.

52. Ibid.

53. Ibid.

54. Ibid.

55. Campbell and Campbell, *The China Study,* 232.

56. Ibid., 228.

57. Ibid., 233.

58. Ibid., 236.

59. Ibid., 164.

60. Ibid., 165.

61. Ibid., 237.

62. Campbell, "Why China Holds the Key to Your Health" published here: http://www.vegsource.com/event/campbell.htm

63. Campbell and Campbell, *The China Study*, 110, 203.

64. Mackey, "Whole Foods Markets' Efforts to Change the World."

65. Ibid.

66. Centers for Disease Control and Prevention, "Body Mass Index," http://www.cdc.gov/healthyweight/assessing/bmi/.

67. Mackey, "Whole Foods Markets' Efforts to Change the World."

68. Barnard, "A Plant-Based Diet for Type-2 Diabetes," Presentation, *McDougall Advanced Lecture Series*, Santa Rosa, CA, February 20, 2010.

CPSIA information can be obtained
at www.ICGtesting.com
Printed in the USA
FSOW04n1132311215
15068FS